6 WAYS
TO LOSE A STONE
IN 6 WEEKS

Judith Wills

Fitness consultant Sarah McClurey

HEADLINE

Copyright © 1998 Judith Wills

Photographs © copyright 1998 Colin Thomas

Jacket photographs:

Diet-testers' 'before' clothes are their own. 'After' clothes supplied by:
Front, l to r: Pam Lawrenson: Debenhams' Jasper Conran jacket, own jeans, Grattan black boots; Guy
Dickens: Debenhams' blue shirt, Grattan jeans, own shoes; Dana Mills: Debenhams' grey long jacket
and skirt, Aristoc tights, Grattan velvet mules.
Back, l to r: Sue Reiss: Debenhams' grey jacket and trousers, Debenhams' coral t-shirt, Littlewoods'
ankle boots; Esther Dickens: Casual Club lilac spaghetti strap t-shirt, Jasper Conran lilac jeans,
Trader mauve velvet-trimmed cardigan (all from Debenhams), Grattan ankle boots; Gareth Dixon:
Debenhams' shirt and tie set, own suit and shoes.

Participants' 'after' clothes styled by Ceril Campbell (0181-780 3088)

The right of Judith Wills to be identified as the Author of the Work has been asserted by her in
accordance with the Copyright, Designs and Patents Act 1988.

First published in 1998 by HEADLINE BOOK PUBLISHING

10 9 8 7 6 5 4 3 2 1

Cataloguing in Publication Data is available from the British Library

ISBN 0 7472 76412

Designed by Isobel Gillan

Typeset by
Letterpart Ltd, Reigate, Surrey

Printed and bound in Italy by
Canale & C. Spa

HEADLINE BOOK PUBLISHING
A division of Hodder Headline PLC
338 Euston Road
London NW1 3BH

6 WAYS
TO LOSE A STONE
IN 6 WEEKS

Judith Wills is one of Britain's best known and most knowledgeable slimming and nutrition experts. Former editor of *Slimmer* magazine, she has also made three bestselling health videos and is an acclaimed cookery writer. Judith bases her writing on sound scientific principles and up-to-date research. Her nutritional advice follows World Health Organisation and Department of Health guidelines and her life as a working mother gives her insight into the problems the average person faces when they try to adopt healthy habits.

She lives in Herefordshire with her husband and two children.

Also by Judith Wills:

Slim for Life

Fat Attack

Size 12 in 21 Days

Take Off Ten Years in Ten Weeks

The Bodysense Diet

100 Favourite Slim and Healthy Recipes

Slim and Healthy Vegetarian

The Food Bible

Contents

introduction

So you want to lose a stone. You're not alone. This is the most usual amount of weight that people do want to lose. Though the media may from time to time give publicity to people who have lost amazing amounts of weight and won prizes and titles for it, for most of us, 10 lb or so – up to two stone – is what we really need to get to grips with. And a stone would do well for 90 per cent of us.

It's also an amount that is easy to put on gradually, without noticing – which is exactly what most of us do. We're not naturally fat or greedy, just preoccupied with other things in life.

It is an amount that doesn't seem **TOO** daunting to lose. It is also an amount that, once lost, has a disproportionately beneficial effect on our looks, our fitness and our self-esteem.

A stone overweight isn't life-threatening or even particularly bad for your health. It's not something to spend sleepless nights over. But most people can think of at least a dozen reasons why they'd prefer that those 14 lb of fat were gone. Looking good in clothes again; getting back into old jeans; being able to try on new clothes in the changing room without feeling embarrassed. A stone or so can represent up to one and a half dress sizes or a 3 inch waistband reduction for men.

On a more serious note, one stone too much **NOW** may be two stones too much in five years' time; three stones too much in ten years' time. And by then, the surplus weight most certainly **CAN** affect your health and fitness, and the length of your life. So to my mind, it makes sense to do something about overweight before it gets too much of a problem.

Six Weeks

So why six weeks to lose a stone? Well, it's the shortest time in which most people can lose a stone within the current recognised guidelines as to what is safe and sensible. 'Up to 2 lb a week' is the mantra for slimmers – an amount that can be lost following a diet that is neither too low in calories or nutrients, and with the help of exercise. Over six weeks this, obviously, comes to 12 lb – but in the first week or two of any slimming plan extra pounds (mostly in the form of a fluid mix called glycogen) are lost.

However, I cannot put my hand on my heart and say categorically that **YOU** will lose exactly a stone in the six weeks, even if you follow one of the plans to the letter. Weight loss depends upon too many factors for me to be able to make such a prediction.

The main factors affecting your final result are:

- If you are very overweight (i.e. you need to lose much more than a stone) you will probably lose more than average. If you are very heavy and you lose more than 10 lb in the first three weeks, you should increase portion sizes slightly and/or have an extra snack a day.
- If you are young you will probably lose more than average. Our metabolic rate slows down slightly as we get older and we are naturally less active.
- If you are apple-shaped rather than pear-shaped you will probably find that the weight comes off more easily. If you are pear-shaped and not very heavy on top, you should be happy with a smaller weight loss, as my participant Sue Rudolf was.
- If you have a scant stone to lose – particularly if you already have a body mass index of 25 or under (see page 13) – and are aiming for a low final weight, you will almost undoubtedly not lose a whole stone in the six weeks. For you it is vital to read Chapters 1 and 2 to make sure that you do really want or need to lose weight.

Other factors, such as prescription drugs, activity levels and so on, will also have a bearing on the exact amount you lose. The amounts my participants lost varied, more or less in accordance with the probabilities above. All I can say is that for many people, a stone or thereabouts in six weeks is possible, if you exercise as well as eat fewer calories. The plans in this book will particularly suit you if you enjoy an allotted time in which to carry out projects; if you enjoy working to a deadline; if you need a strong motivation to get you moving; and if you need to see real results in order to keep motivation up.

There are six different plans to cover most lifestyles and preferences. Use Chapter 1 to help you decide which is the right one for you at this time and don't even consider beginning a plan until you've read Chapters 1 and 2 thoroughly. Keep the book on your shelf even when you've shed your weight because it is full of tips, recipes, and so on that will help you maintain your weight in the years ahead.

Throughout the book you will find photographs and 'case histories' of some of the people who tested out these programmes for you. I found my participants simply by placing a small ad in a newspaper and was amazed at the huge response that ad brought. You will, I hope, find their comments, photos and stories further motivation to begin a plan yourself. As you will see, they didn't all find it exactly **EASY** – particularly the exercise, in some cases – but they were all thrilled to see their new figures taking shape, and have been honest about the bad times as well as the good. I think one of the most interesting points to emerge from their 'test runs' was that most of them went on holiday during the six weeks, all led busy lives, had friends round, dined out – and still managed to succeed.

If you need any more motivation to begin, pick up a couple of bags of shopping that add up to a stone – and think of that extra weight on your body. The time has come. The advice is here. **DO IT!**

so you want to lose a stone (or so)?

If there are approximately 14 lb between you and the body you want – or, probably, the body you used to have! – then there is no need to allow the weight to linger any longer. You **CAN** do something about it. And now is as good a time as any to start.

This book shows how to get down to a reasonable weight for you – and how to stay there. But first, in this chapter, we need to look at how your surplus poundage got there, why it is bothering you so much, and what you need to know and do before actually beginning your slimming and shape-up plan.

Just how did that stone get there?

Before you consider losing a stone, it will be useful first to look at the reasons that this amount of excess weight may have accumulated on your body. Looking at these factors will help us to see what is needed to get it off again. And it is also a good starting place for you to be totally honest with yourself (if, by any chance, you, like many people, have tended to fantasise somewhat about life and its relationship with your body shape and weight – as, for example, 'I hardly eat a thing – how can I have put on a stone since I got married?').

It probably got there slowly

Very few people pile on a stone in weeks – it is more likely to have arrived insidiously, so gradually that you hardly noticed until you had to go up a waistband size or two and suddenly one day realised that you no longer feel good in swimwear on the beach.

The fact is that overeating by a very small amount on a regular basis is enough to put on a few pounds a year. 'Overeating' doesn't mean pigging out, going on massive chocolate, bread or cheese binges, and so on. All 'overeating' means is eating or drinking more calories than your body needs to maintain its reasonable weight. Your threshold may be different from someone else's (see Chapter 2 for answers to sticky questions such as 'Is it my genes?'), but if you've been eating, for example, just two biscuits a day or one glass of wine a day more in terms of calories than your body needs (each of which are about 100 calories a day) then totted up over a year that represents a weight gain of 10 lb or so a year. As another example, one typical restaurant three-course meal with wine (about 2,000 calories) indulged in once a fortnight for a year without cutting back a little on what you eat in other areas could put on about 7 lb in that year.

The point of mentioning that most surplus weight comes on slowly and is very easy to put on is to make you understand that most of you aren't self-indulgent, slobby, piggy people with weak willpower and no sense of pride. You are quite normal, with normal appetite and lifestyle. And, as such, you should stop feeling guilty about what you perceive as your 'weight problem'.

It **ISN'T A PROBLEM** – it is just surplus weight (if, indeed, it **IS** surplus to requirements – a discussion which we will be coming to in a minute) and you aren't a sinner for having gained it. But you should be in no doubt that if you are genuinely a stone or so overweight then it **IS** because you have eaten 'surplus to requirements' over a period of time. OK, maybe someone else could eat what you eat and not put on an ounce – that is a fact – but that's not the point. Again, Chapter 2 should clear up all the questions you may have on the unfairness of food, weight and slimming.

It probably started to come on when you made lifestyle changes

When did weight gain begin for you?

Maybe you got married or began a live-in relationship. You had a baby, or two. You took a new job that involved lots of entertaining or sessions in the wine bar. Or perhaps your new job involved less leg work and more desk work.

It could be you split up with a partner and began couch-potato evenings with wine and chocolates for company. It could be you left college and stopped your regular sports sessions.

Putting on weight is almost always involved with your lifestyle, a lifestyle which means that you eat more calories than you need and/or burn off too few through exercise.

I mention this because it is very hard to lose weight and keep it off unless you recognise these lifestyle-related weight-gain opportunities. Once recognised, there are two ways you can go. You may decide to find ways to lose weight while keeping your current lifestyle (e.g. you're not going to stop being a couch potato but you'll drink diet Coke and nibble on fruit instead). Or you may prefer to go the whole hog, and change your lifestyle (e.g. you switch off the telly and go for a brisk walk) – a solution which is often the harder of the two initially but may, long term, be easier.

Whichever way you decide to play it, this book offers a variety of programmes to suit. The questionnaire at the end of this chapter will help you to decide whether you want to make subtle or radical changes to your lifestyle, then lead to the right programme for you.

It came on because too many people want you to overeat

Your spare tyre is not there because you tried one diet too many in your past. (What nonsense!) It is there, as I have already mentioned, because you have been eating more than your body needs for fuel. When you do that, surplus calories in what you eat and drink are then deposited in your body's fat cells.

As we've seen, your lifestyle plays a big part in overweight. But there is another culprit and that culprit is, collectively, the modern food industry. Billions of pounds every year are spent on food, drinks, snacks and edibles (if you like to call them so) that our bodies don't need. We get fat on food surplus to requirements. And in turn, the food industry gets fat on the profits from these gigantic mountains of unnecessary calories that it puts into our mouths.

The food manufacturers and major sellers do not want us to be slim. And so they are not sitting there idly hoping that we will eat and eat, and fill their coffers. They are permanently busy **PERSUADING** us to eat (and spending billions of pounds a year on doing so).

Persuading us through advertising – both up front on TV, in magazines, and so on, and also in more subtle ways, such as by sponsorships (even in schools – get them young!), and in the sheer size of the packages of food that are produced (multipacks, 'extra free' packs and so on). If you want a tin of baked beans or a can of lager, it is hard to get just one these days. You have to buy big.

Persuading us through temptation (crisps or chocolate bought at the newspaper counter on impulse) – and through a hundred other ways. The food industry wants you to buy, buy, buy.

And, as every food addict knows, if it's bought, you eat it. Not because you need it, but because it is there.

This is, largely (excuse the pun), how you got overweight. And if you want to slim and stay slim, you need to become permanently aware of the fact that you're often eating not because **YOU** want to – but because someone else wants you to. If you still need persuading that I am not exaggerating, think on this – if everyone in the UK who needed to lose a stone actually did so, I estimate that this would be equivalent to 500 billion calories uneaten and would represent about £490 billion in lost revenue to the food industry!

A major solution to losing weight and keeping it off is to train yourself to recognise each and every occasion when you are eating or drinking because of these powers of persuasion at work, and not because you really want to or need to eat and drink. You also need to recognise that the **TYPE** of food you are eating and drinking is largely influenced by the food industry. There is little profit to be made in unadulterated, natural foods compared with the profit that there is to be made from what the industry calls 'added value' foods (highly processed, highly promoted foods, often 'treat' foods). Which is why

you don't often see carrots advertised on TV. You think you can't live without a hefty daily dose of junk food or fat or sweets. I think that you can – and that you would be surprised how easily you can.

We all need to eat, we all need to shop, we all want to use the convenience of the supermarket. But use **THEM** – don't let them use you, and your expanding waistline, to make a profit.

And while on the subject of persuasion, it is worth mentioning that your own family, friends, colleagues and so on can also do quite a good job of getting you to eat when you don't really want or need to – so it is worth developing your ability to say the word 'no' to them, as well.

Why is losing just a stone so hard to do?

The answers to the previous question have largely answered this question too. Your lifestyle and the modern commercial world that we live in sometimes seem like a conspiracy to keep you overweight. Previous attempts to diet may have failed because the diets didn't supply you with enough ammunition to overcome the problems. To alter the balance in your favour and succeed this time, you need to:

A   know what made you fat;
B   take control and responsibility for your diet, knowing when to say 'no' and when to say 'yes'; and
C   learn new habits to replace the old 'fat' habits – entailing subtle or radical changes.

(A) we have already discussed. (B) and (C) are not hard to do as long as your motivation to change your tactics, and your need and desire to lose weight are both stronger than your inclination to carry on as before. Below we look at ways to stoke up your motivation levels so that this time you **WILL** achieve success.

A few other factors that may strongly affect your ability to lose a stone or so need mentioning first, though.

Exercise

As a stone overweight isn't a great deal overweight, every little way you can increase your daily calorie 'deficit' to encourage your body to burn off its own fat is important. Exercise burns up calories and therefore is very important. If you've tried to diet before without exercising – take it from me, don't try again. You need to increase your activity levels. I know many of you hate exercise – which is why I have devoted a whole chapter to it later in the book, and why I have called it the 'E' word!

Duff diets

If you've tried, and failed, to stick to a variety of diets in the past, the main reason will have been that those particular diets weren't right for you. If you want slimming to fit in with your current lifestyle, you need the diet to do that, and not you to adapt to the diet too much. If you're prepared to make lifestyle changes, you need a diet plan that matches your ideas on what you want to achieve: better health, well-being, fitness, and so on, and that is a good basis for a diet for life. Many diets aren't.

Socialising

Eating out, entertaining, going on holiday, Christmas, birthdays – one of the main problems I hear from would-be slimmers is that they can't lose weight because they lead too busy a social/business life. Yes, this does make life more difficult, but it can be overcome (as we prove in Chapter 7).

Maybe you don't really need to lose a stone

When I have been talking about losing a stone, I have assumed that you really do need to lose a stone. But there are a lot of people who think they do need to lose weight when in fact they don't; they are fine as they are. For such people, losing weight is hard and if they do manage to take off a few pounds or more, it soon comes back. Moral – if you try for too low a body weight, your life will probably be one long and miserable round of weight loss and weight gain, or eating like a sparrow to stay thin.

I don't want you to be thin. I want you to be a comfortable and reasonable body weight. After we've discussed motivation, we'll take a close look at your current weight, your weight target – and whether or not you really do need to shed 14 lb or so.

Why does a surplus stone matter anyway?

I have to assume that if you are looking at this book you do feel as though you want to lose a stone. You will not be reading it if you are fat and happy, unless you happen to be a book critic. But **WHY** do you want to lose a stone?

If you arm yourself with a huge list of reasons why, you stand a greater chance of success. Motivation is the key. So let's look at all the many reasons you could consider.

Looks

From talking to the people who followed this programme, and have followed other slimming programmes of mine, I believe that both men and women want to lose weight for vanity's sake – to look better, and to have a better choice of clothes.

I see nothing wrong with a bit of vanity – too many overweight people lack self-confidence, and slimming down and being able to wear gorgeous, figure-hugging dresses or a tight pair of jeans is just the boost they need.

Although it is wrong, all research shows that employers, given a choice of a fat person and a slimmer person with the same qualifications, will choose the slimmer person. Appearances do matter.

When you're truly overweight, you may lose your waistline, have a fat belly, a double chin, flabby upper arms, bum and thighs. Your cheekbones will disappear and whatever the makers of larger-size clothes may say, clothes just don't hang right on a big figure.

At a genuine stone overweight, you may still look all right in what you wear – but give it a few more years and a few more stones, and you probably won't.

Health

At a genuine stone overweight, you are unlikely to be suffering from health problems connected with your weight. But all the evidence shows that most people gradually pile on more and more weight over the years unless they choose to do something about it. A stone now, given a few more years, will be two or three stones and your Body Mass Index (see next section) will creep towards the unacceptable, giving rise to all kinds of health problems such as increased risk of high blood pressure, heart disease, arthritis, diabetes and so on. If your surplus weight is concentrated around your waist, the health risks are greatest.

The 'fat is fine' lobby, with champions such as Dawn French and Vanessa Feltz, will tell you that they are perfectly fit and healthy and that a lot of rot is talked about overweight and health. In America, where over 50 per cent of the population is now overweight, the 'fat is fine' lobby is very strong. But, despite that, the US Government has just rewritten the official guidelines on correct weight for height.

And they've rewritten them **DOWN**, not up – because the link between overweight, ill health and shortened lifespan isn't a myth, it's proven fact.

You want good health and a long life, don't you? You don't want to be 60 and having trouble walking up a gentle incline, or getting up a flight of stairs? If you can avoid angina, diabetes, painful hips and knee joints, and various other niggling problems as you get older – you would prefer to do so, wouldn't you?

In that case, you need to watch your weight. If you're a stone or so overweight now – lose it, or see it increase.

Feelings

I mentioned the increased sense of confidence that comes from being a reasonable weight. If you slim as I suggest, increasing your activity levels and eating a healthy diet, you will not only look better (from most people's perspective) but also feel better, too, in many ways.

Many overweight people complain of feeling lethargic – almost every person I have helped to slim says they feel much more energetic, alive, happy and alert. This is mostly due to the exercise but is also a result of feeling good about themselves and their achievement.

Many overweight people feel guilty and/or angry, and/or annoyed about their eating habits and about not being able to control them or their weight. As I've explained, being fat is not really your fault, but once you've understood the reasons, it **IS** your responsibility to get on with it, overcome the factors making you overeat or lead a sedentary lifestyle, and take control. Lose that weight and you kill the burden of guilt and anger too. It's a tonic you deserve.

Many overweight people spend hours and hours every day thinking about their size and their weight. Two hours a day spent on negative thought and no action is equal to six and a quarter years of your life wasted. And yet one of the main excuses I hear from people who say they want to lose weight but aren't managing it is that they 'don't have time'. They do have time, if they want to find it. Anyway, it really doesn't take any more time to eat a sensible slimming diet than it does to eat a load of food you don't need, as the Healthy Fast Food Plan demonstrates. Lose the weight, get your eating and activity habits under control and you need spend no more time worrying about it all.

o   o   o

Before we go any further, it would be a good idea to draw up your own list of reasons why you want to lose a stone or so. Done? Are they enough motivation?

Ask yourself:

- Do I really want to do this?
- Am I prepared to make the necessary changes to my diet and/or lifestyle?
- Am I prepared to agree that if I really want to lose weight I can find the time in my life to do what it takes?
- Am I prepared to agree that good diet and good exercise are a priority in my life?
- Do I agree that some of what I have been eating is unnecessary for my body needs?

Do you really need to lose weight?

Before beginning any slimming programme it is wise, both for your sanity's sake and your health's sake, to check that you are actually overweight. Quite a lot of people I see (especially women) think they are fat when they are not. Sometimes they just need to firm up their 'flabby bits' in order to look more

streamlined; other times they are being unrealistic – often people in their forties and fifties want to get back to a very low weight that they were in their late teens or early twenties, when research shows that it is healthier, as you get older, to be an 'average' weight rather than very slim.

The point about weight is that it isn't an exact science – there is plenty of flexibility about what constitutes a reasonable weight for a particular height. Two women of the same height and age can vary in their respective weights by two stone or so, and still both be within a healthy weight range.

Unless you were an overweight child/teenager, most people tend to use as a yardstick their weight in their early twenties. As we've seen, this may be too low a weight for you if you are now 40-plus and so, when considering what your target weight should be, you should add on about 3 lb for every 10 years older than 20 that you are, up to the age of 60.

For example, if you are aged 50, 5ft 5ins and weighed 9 stone at 20, a more realistic and sensible target would be a minimum of 9 stone 9lbs.

On page 15 there is a height/weight chart which is based on the Body Mass Index – an internationally accepted index used by professionals. This index is worked out by taking a person's weight in kilograms and dividing it by their squared height (in metres). The resulting figure is that person's BMI, and the classification for BMIs is as follows:

- Below 20 – underweight (may cause health problems).
- Between 20 and 25 – acceptable weight range.
- Between 25 and 30 – overweight (may cause health problems especially if towards top of this range).
- Between 30 and 40 – obese (increased likelihood of weight-related health problems and mortality).
- Over 40 – extremely obese (high likelihood of weight-related health problems and early death).

The height/weight chart opposite shows lower and upper weight limits based loosely on the BMI range of 20–25. In fact, my 'lowest weights to aim for' in the first weight column work out at a BMI slightly over 20 (in the region of 20.5), because, as I said earlier, I don't want you to be thin, or very slim, call it what you will.

My 'highest acceptable weights' in the second weight column work out, again, at a BMI slightly higher than 25 (but only slightly), as, depending upon your natural shape and where the weight lies, there is some room for manoeuvre here.

Weigh yourself and compare your own weight for height with the lower and upper limits in the chart.

- If you are at or near the lower limit – don't bother trying to lose weight; you don't need to.
- If you are about midway between the two, your BMI is around 22.5–23, and near enough perfect. If you still think you are overweight, ask yourself, 'Do I simply need to tone up? Am I being unrealistic?'
- If your weight is near or at the upper limit, then cosmetically, you may wish to slim down a stone or so to bring your BMI nearer the acceptable average of 22.5–23. It has been discovered that males live longest and are healthiest if they have a BMI of around 22. There are no available statistics for women, but because women tend to have a higher body-fat percentage than men, my estimate is that a BMI of 23 is ideal for women. Roughly speaking, a weight halfway between the lower limit and the upper limit (for any particular height) on my chart is a BMI of 22.5. Remember, the lower you aim below your comfortable weight, the harder it will be for you to keep the weight off for good.
- If your weight is much over the upper limit, then you are right to want to lose weight. You should at first set your target at, or near, that upper limit and then assess yourself again when you have slimmed down to the upper limit given.

Your final reasonable body weight will depend upon various factors, including:

Your own preferences

Aim for a weight at which you feel comfortable. But if you have been very overweight (and maybe, for a long time), an average weight rather than a very slim weight would be more sensible.

Your body-fat distribution

Many health professionals are now inclined to set more store by a person's waist circumference than they are by weight. This is because research has shown that the size of your waist can directly predict health problems such as high blood pressure and heart disease.

If you are male and your waist measurement is between 94cm and 101cm, or female and your waist is between 80cm and 87cm, you are $1\frac{1}{2}$ times more likely to have major heart problems.

If you are male and your waist measurement is over 101cm, or female and it is over 87cm, the risk increases to between $2\frac{1}{2}$ and $4\frac{1}{2}$ times.

In other words, if you tend to carry your fat around your middle (rather than on your hips and thighs, chest or elsewhere) you may need to slim down to a lower BMI (but still within the 20–25 guidelines) than other people who are, say, pear-shaped, in order to get your waistline into shape. Measure your waist and let this help you decide. If your waist is under 94cm (male) or 80cm (female) then you needn't slim for health reasons.

Your age

The older you are the less you should consider trying to slim to à BMI of under 22. If you are still not sure whether or not you should lose weight, or what your initial target should be, visit your doctor or health centre dietician. There is more information on sensible slimming and weight control in the next chapter.

Height/weight chart for men and women

Based on the Body Mass Index charts

Height (without shoes)	Weight (without clothes)	
	Lower limit (roughly equivalent to BMI 20.5)	Upper limit (roughly equivalent to BMI 25)
5 ft	7 st 4 lb	8 st 12 lb
5 ft 1 in	7 st 7 lb	9 st 3 lb
5 ft 2 in	7 st 10 lb	9 st 6 lb
5 ft 3 in	8 st 0 lb	9 st 11 lb
5 ft 4 in	8 st 4 lb	10 st 2 lb
5 ft 5 in	8 st 8 lb	10 st 6 lb
5 ft 6 in	8 st 11 lb	10 st 11 lb
5 ft 7 in	9 st 1 lb	11 st 2 lb
5 ft 8 in	9 st 5 lb	11 st 7 lb
5 ft 9 in	9 st 8 lb	11 st 12 lb
5 ft 10 in	9 st 13 lb	12 st 3 lb
5 ft 11 in	10 st 3 lb	12 st 8 lb
6 ft	10 st 7 lb	12 st 13 lb
6 ft 1 in	10 st 11 lb	13 st 4 lb
6 ft 2 in	11 st 1 lb	13 st 9 lb
6 ft 3 in	11 st 5 lb	14 st 0 lb

Six ways to lose a stone – which one is right for you?

Chapters 3 to 8 offer six different slimming programmes to help you lose a stone or so.

They are the Detox and Energise Plan, the Healthy Fast Food Plan, the Sweet-tooth Plan, the Meat-free Plan, the Business Plan and the Family Plan. If you are not sure which of the plans is right for you at this time, use the following questionnaire to help you decide. Simply answer the six sets of questions and add up your 'yes' answers for each set, then see for which set you have most often answered 'yes'. This then is probably your favoured plan.

Detox and Energise

	Yes	No
Do you feel below par, lacking in energy, run down?	☐	☐
Do you feel that your diet is unhealthy, with too many high-fat, high-sugar, high-salt and processed products?	☐	☐
Do you feel like making a new beginning?	☐	☐
Will your lifestyle allow you to eat plenty of fresh food *or* are you prepared to change your lifestyle and place more emphasis on healthy diet?	☐	☐
Are you happy to eat little meat and animal produce?	☐	☐
Do you tend to get digestive problems, perhaps including bloating, constipation, fluid retention?	☐	☐
Is good health one of your main motivators for slimming?	☐	☐
Do you enjoy the idea of simplicity and minimalism within your diet?	☐	☐

Healthy Fast Food

	Yes	No
Do you lead a very busy lifestyle which you feel unable to change?	☐	☐
Do you rely a lot on convenience meals and fast food?	☐	☐
Do you resent time spent cooking?	☐	☐
Have you found on any previous attempts to lose weight that you had to give up because healthy reduced-calorie food seemed too time-consuming?	☐	☐
Are you happy to eat 'little and often'?	☐	☐
Do you live alone, or, at least, require meals just for yourself?	☐	☐
Are you happy to pay a little extra for healthy fast food?	☐	☐
Do you enjoy a wide variety of foods?	☐	☐

Sweet-tooth

	Yes	No
Do you like chocolate and/or confectionery?	☐	☐
Do you like puddings and desserts?	☐	☐
Do you like biscuits, cakes and other sweet snacks?	☐	☐
Do you like the idea of incorporating sweet foods into a healthy slimming plan?	☐	☐
Would you like to learn how to control the urge to overindulge in sweet foods?	☐	☐
Do you like a wide variety of other foods?	☐	☐
Would you call yourself an organised person?	☐	☐
Are you prepared to accept that you can't lose weight steadily unless you are prepared to modify your diet to include sweet foods in reasonable but not excessive quantities?	☐	☐

Meat-free

	Yes	No
If currently a meat-eater, have you lately been considering going vegetarian or demi-vegetarian (fish only)?	☐	☐
Are you vegetarian or demi-vegetarian?	☐	☐
Do you like cooking (as long as it's not too time-consuming or difficult)?	☐	☐
Would you like to increase your fruit, vegetable and salad intake?	☐	☐
Would you like to increase your fibre intake?	☐	☐
Would you like to cut down on your saturated fat intake and on your overall fat intake?	☐	☐
Is there any history of heart disease and/or cancer in your family?	☐	☐
Have you tried to lose weight before and found it hard?	☐	☐

Business

	Yes	No
Do you have a demanding career?	☐	☐
Do you have to eat out a lot?	☐	☐
Do you have to entertain a lot?	☐	☐
Do you think you are drinking too much alcohol?	☐	☐
Do you find your eating patterns erratic (missing meals, grabbing what's handy)?	☐	☐
Do you find there is often little time to plan meals, shop or think about food?	☐	☐
Do you get home late, hungry, with little suitable to eat?	☐	☐
Would you be prepared to spend a little time every weekend (approx. I hour) organising your diet?	☐	☐

Family

	Yes	No
Do you have a family/partner?	☐	☐
Do you tend to want main meals that the family can share, at least most of the time?	☐	☐
Do you want to avoid preparing separate meals for yourself?	☐	☐
Is budget an important factor in what you buy?	☐	☐
Do you (or your partner) enjoy cooking simple, tasty meals that aren't too time-consuming?	☐	☐
Does the family enjoy a range of meals – from traditional roasts to stir-fries and curries?	☐	☐
Would you like to learn how to cut fat and calories in ordinary, everyday meals?	☐	☐
Does anyone else in the family need to lose weight?	☐	☐

top ten slimming questions

- and the Truthful Answers

1. How quickly can I safely lose weight?

The recommendation generally given by health professionals is that optimal weight loss is up to 2 lb a week on a varied, healthy reduced-calorie diet. Faster weight loss than this means that more lean body tissue, from muscles and organs, will be lost. Fast weight loss due to a very low-calorie diet may also mean inadequate intake of nutrients such as the complete range of vitamins and minerals, protein and essential fats, and some research indicates that people who lose weight too quickly are more likely to regain that weight.

However, in the first week or two of any reduced-calorie diet, there will be extra weight loss, in the form of body fluid and glycogen (a mixture of glucose and other body fluids), due to the decrease in the amount of calories and carbohydrate being eaten. (Carbohydrate tends to act a bit like a sponge in the body, helping it to retain more fluid. When carbohydrate intake is reduced, a proportion of this fluid is excreted and shows on the scales as weight loss. After one to two weeks, weight loss will no longer include a glycogen factor but be a mixture of body fat and lean tissue.)

Thus if you need to lose a stone, in theory you could safely lose it in around six weeks (2 lb a week × 6 = 12 lb, plus an extra 2–3 lb of body fluid). This is the minimum time you should allow.

That is the broad theory of what the 'average' person can do. However, there are many variables and these need to be discussed here.

How much overweight you are

Generally speaking, the more overweight you are at the start of your slimming plan, the easier it will be for you to lose weight steadily at 2 lb a week. Indeed, if you are very overweight, with a BMI of, say, more than 30, you should be able to eat much more than the calorie levels that appear in the plans in this book and still lose 2 lb a week.

On the other hand, if you are only a little overweight – say, within the acceptable BMI range – at the start of slimming, it is probably unrealistic to expect weight loss of 2 lb a week. (Indeed, as we saw in Chapter 1, if you already have a BMI of 25 or below, you may not need to lose weight at all.) Therefore as a rough guide, the less weight you want to lose, the slower it will probably come off.

What your target weight is

If you want to lose a stone to bring your BMI down to 25 (see explanation of BMI and upper limit for your height, chart on page 15), you will probably find losing 2 lb a week easier than if you want to lose a stone to bring your BMI down to the 20–23 range. In other words, the lower you set your target weight, the slower it will probably come off. The moral here – don't set your target weight unrealistically low!

Your body shape

If you are 'apple-shaped' (see Chapter 1) with most of your surplus poundage around your tummy and waist, then you will probably find the pounds easier to lose than a 'pear-shaped' person, with their weight around the hips and thighs. As we saw in Chapter 1, pear-shaped people, who in theory register as overweight on the scales, may be perfectly healthy and in no need of slimming at all. It is recognised that 'pear' weight is harder to shift, and an overweight 'pear' should probably be happy with a weight loss of less than 2 lb a week, and set a BMI target of no less than 23.

Your height

Taller people often find that the weight comes off more easily than short people. That is probably because, pro rata, smaller people have less to lose and need to eat less than tall people in order to lose weight at the same rate. (The reason for this is that small people need fewer calories in daily living than tall people do, because there isn't so much body mass to energise and service. Therefore small people also need fewer calories on a diet, to create an adequate calorie deficit. But rather than exist on too few calories, it is better for small people to lose weight more slowly.)

Your age

Young people are more likely to lose weight at 2 lb a week than older people following a similar diet. That is because our metabolic rate slows down with age (see Question 8), albeit slowly. If we don't exercise and keep our muscle mass as intact as possible, it may slow down faster. To lose weight at the same rate as a young person of the same weight and height, an older person would usually need to eat less – this may not be a good idea and so to be content with slower weight loss may be the sensible answer.

Your activity levels

The more calories you burn up through activity, both formal and informal, the greater the calorie deficit you are creating. If a previously inactive person begins regular exercise to burn up an extra, say, 250 calories a day, then in theory that person would lose ½ lb a week even without eating fewer calories.

Combining a sensible reduction in calorie intake with a reasonable increase in energy expenditure is recognised to be the best way to lose weight.

All these factors must be considered when you think about losing weight. To lose a stone in six weeks, and/or to lose 2 lb a week mid or long term on any diet, is the **MAXIMUM** recommended. If many of the factors listed above which may slow down your weight loss apply to you, then you should be happy to lose weight at 1 lb a week, setting a realistic target weight.

A loss of 6 lb in six weeks is not to be sneezed at. You can follow any of the diets in this book and even if you don't lose 2 lb a week you should still consider yourself a success. You can carry on with any of the diets for more weeks until you do reach your own reasonable weight, if necessary.

Another point to consider is your own temperament. Some people will never lose weight unless they see a noticeable improvement in their waistline, or on the scales, quite quickly. Some people enjoy setting themselves targets and 'going for it'. If that sounds like you, then structured programmes such as those in this book are for you.

Other people don't like to feel pressured in any way and may find that by simply adopting a few changes in their current diet over a period of months or longer, they gradually lose weight. Some experts say this is the only sensible way to lose weight, and for long-term 'yo-yo' dieters (see Question 6), this may be the preferred method.

I can see both points of view, and feel that there is room for both approaches to weight loss.

Perhaps at the end of the day we should recognise that it isn't so much getting genuine surplus weight off that is important, but learning how to keep it off.

I hope that the plans in this book will help everyone to do that, whether you manage 2 lb a week or whether the weight comes off more slowly.

NOTE If you are pregnant, breast feeding, ill, convalescing or with any special medical condition, it is important not to attempt any slimming diet or exercise without consulting your physician.

2. Can I spot reduce my problem areas through diet?

No, not really. When you reduce your calorie intake, there is no way that you can tell your body fat to disappear from certain areas and not from others – it isn't listening! Though because of the way weight sometimes tends to be distributed, it may seem to you as though spot reduction is happening. For example, if you are an 'apple' shape, with much of your surplus weight around your middle, you may be

pleased to find that your spare tyre begins disappearing in a very well-behaved manner shortly after you start the diet. This is because centrally distributed body fat does shift more easily than fat elsewhere on the body. If you are a woman, it may also go quite rapidly from your bust; but the fat on your thighs, calves and ankles will take much longer to disappear. Hip and thigh fat on women is a much more durable type of fat and **IS** harder to shift; though if it really is surplus to requirements it **WILL** improve with diet and exercise.

And that last word, exercise, is the key to so-called 'spot reduction'. You can't call the shots about where the fat goes from through diet – but you **CAN** call most of the shots when it comes to toning up your muscles.

Many of us who think we need a diet in fact need nothing more than better muscle tone. A fat tummy can be 'slimmed' with good abdominal exercise. A flabby bum can be turned firm and round with regular gluteal exercise – and so on.

That is why, if you want your body to look and feel in its best shape, you do need to exercise. And that is especially true once you pass 30. Left to its own devices, after 30 your body, at first slowly, begins to bow to gravity. Give it some regular help, and you can keep looking slim and toned.

It has been estimated that you can **LOOK** up to a stone slimmer without shedding an ounce – just through toning exercise. For more on exercise, see Chapter 9.

3. How do I avoid hunger when I'm slimming?

If there is one thing that most of us fear about a slimming programme, it is the thought of hunger. More than chocolate deprivation, more than taste deprivation. We hate to feel hungry!

In fact, true hunger isn't necessary on any slimming diet. Show me any high-calorie meal, and I can show you a plateful of food, similar in style, that actually weighs more yet contains about half the calories.

The key to no-hunger is eating the right types of food at the right times. If you've been ravenous on past slimming attempts, let's look at some of the possible reasons why.

Calorie content too low

If a 16-stone man tries to follow a diet aimed at an average woman with a few pounds to lose, he will feel hungry. If an average woman with a few pounds to lose tries to live on three milk-shake replacement meals a day, she will feel hungry. Moral – tailor your diet to yourself. As a rule of thumb, a woman will need 1,250–1,500 calories a day, based on a nutritionally sound diet, if she isn't to feel hungry, and a man 1,400–1,700.

Wrong types of food

1,250 calories a day of cake and sweets, pies, pastries and highly processed food will leave most average women slimmers feeling hungry, but 1,250 calories a day of a variety of wholesome foods including lean proteins, carbohydrates, fresh fruits and vegetables, won't.

There are two reasons for this.

First, because much sweet and 'junk' food is high in calories, you don't get much food for your calorie allowance. As an example, 1,250 calories a day could be used up with nothing more than one medium slice of sponge cake and three chocolate bars. Used wisely, it can provide a breakfast, a lunch, an evening meal and two small snacks.

Secondly, a poor diet tends to contain more foods which are high on what is called the Glycaemic Index. This is a chart used by dieticians to measure the rate

at which carbohydrate foods are absorbed into the bloodstream. A food with a high GI is rapidly absorbed; a food with a low GI is slowly absorbed. Low GI foods, such as many vegetables, fruits, wholegrain cereals and pulses, keep the blood sugar levels more even throughout the day and will help keep hunger pangs at bay. So to avoid hunger, each meal or snack should contain some low GI food.

Although the Glycaemic Index applies only to carbohydrate foods and not to proteins and fats, both protein and fat have the same effect as low GI foods.

Therefore, the best hunger-prevention diet is one that is high in low GI foods and contains a little protein and fat at every meal/snack. The diets in this book all take advantage of this fact and thus help to prevent you feeling hungry.

Meals not eaten frequently enough

Many slimmers try to exist on one meal a day. This takes strong willpower and in fact isn't the ideal way to slim at all. Several small meals and snacks a day are a much better idea. Little and often, like low GI foods, helps keep the blood sugar levels even and helps to prevent hunger.

Bland diet containing foods unappealing to you

Much hunger is psychological and one great cause of this 'pretend' hunger is that your mouth, your nose and your tastebuds aren't getting a good enough 'workout' on your diet. You need strong tastes, appetising aromas, plenty to chew on and plenty of colourful foods on your plate to make you feel satisfied.

Cottage cheese and a few lettuce leaves never did do much for many slimmers!

Meals to suit the clock and not your own hunger patterns

Many slimmers eat by the clock and not when they are beginning to feel hungry. Successful slimmers tend to get in touch with their own 'hungry times of day' and eat to suit that. For an example, many people have a lunch around 1pm and try to wait until, say, 7.30pm before having an evening meal. And yet most people say to me that one of their hungriest times of day is around 5–6pm. A later lunch, plus a small snack at 5pm would be a much more sensible idea.

4. Why does weight loss slow down or stop after I've been slimming for some time, and how can I prevent this?

As we saw in Question 1, anyone who begins a weight loss programme will lose more weight in the first week or two of a diet due to glycogen and fluid loss. Weight loss should then slow down and an average of 2 lb a week loss is nowadays considered very good.

However, few people will lose exactly 2 lb – no more, no less – every week. Loss will fluctuate. In women this may be due to hormonal changes, for example in the monthly cycle (a gain of 3 lb fluid before a period is normal – this will disappear after the period begins). Carbohydrate intake may vary from day to day and this will alter the balance of fluid in the body.

But, on a long-term diet, it is quite normal for weight loss gradually to slow down. This is because the nearer you get to target weight, the slower your metabolic rate is. (A person burns up more calories at 12 stone, say, than he or she will at 10 stone, simply because the greater amount of weight means that the body has more work to do.)

The only way to continue to lose weight at the initial rate would be to reduce the calorie content of the diet even more, and/or to increase the amount of exercise done.

In practice, if you are on a reduced-calorie diet it is not a good idea to drop below about 1,250 (see Question 1), so the only scope for reducing the calorie content of the diet would be if your starting calorie level was higher than that, which it would be if your starting weight was very high and you had a lot to lose.

So if you are reaching target weight on a 1,250 (or thereabouts) calorie diet, the main option is to increase exercise **OR** simply to be happy with slower weight loss.

But if weight loss has stopped altogether, the most obvious reason is that you are getting a bit more careless with your diet – either forgetting to count certain drinks, snacks, etc., or unwittingly increasing portion sizes of the higher calorie items. A last reason could be that you were aiming for too low a body weight and that you are slim enough.

5. Is there really any miracle way to lose weight without dieting?

You can lose body fat with the surgical procedure liposuction, which is costly, often painful and has mixed results.

You can lose pounds of fluid by sweating, e.g. through vigorous exercise wearing warm clothes, or in a sauna or similar. But that weight is just fluid which will return when you drink.

You can go to a doctor who may prescribe slimming pills to speed up your metabolic rate or to dampen your appetite or prevent fat absorption, but I would not recommend this as a course of action for most people as slimming pills can be addictive and have side effects.

You may also be tempted by advertisements you may see in the press offering 'miracle' pills containing all kinds of bizarre ingredients for fabulous weight loss almost overnight without dieting. I'm afraid these are more or less 100 per cent cons.

No – I'm sorry, I really don't know any foolproof, safe, miracle way to lose weight without creating an energy deficit within your body so that it burns off its own fat for fuel. That means eating fewer calories and, if you're sensible, exercising more.

6. Is it true that previous 'yo-yo' dieting could have permanently slowed down my metabolism?

You will read this often in magazines, books and papers. However, I don't know of any actual scientific evidence to show this. The only proper scientific research that has been done on the subject, to my knowledge, was at the Dunn Clinical Nutrition Centre in Cambridge and their results actually disproved this theory. They found that people who 'yo-yo' dieted did no damage to their metabolic rates whatsoever.

In my own experience, I have put many women in their forties and fifties who have spent years 'yo-yo' dieting, on sensible diet and exercise regimes and most have succeeded in losing weight at a reasonable rate without pain, and in keeping it off.

I would say that if you have been a typical 'yo-yoer' in the past, don't let that put you off trying again. The main thing to remember is to take regular exercise and to be happy with a maximum weight loss of 2 lb a week, to follow a varied, nutritious and sensible diet, and to think long term of food as enjoyable, rather than something you battle with all the time. You should also go back to Chapter 1 and Question 1 in this chapter and take on board the importance of a sensible weight target and type of diet.

In other words, I am quite sure that the reason 'yo-yo' dieters have trouble keeping their weight off is not because their metabolisms are wrecked, but for lifestyle and psychological reasons.

7. Why is it that however little I eat, I can't lose weight?

There have been one or two famous studies which have proved, conclusively, that normal, healthy, overweight women fed on 1,000-calorie-a-day diets always lose weight. A thousand calories a day is now considered too low a dieting level for most people, but it still represents a lot more food than some people say they eat and still can't lose any weight. This means that such people think they are eating less than they really are.

A diet high in fats and sugars can seem quite little because these are dense foods that don't look much on the plate or in the hand. Other people forget about the calories in drink – even a glass of orange juice may contain 100 calories.

Most overweight people can lose weight quite well on 1,500 calories a day; 1,250 is a minimum calorie level. So if you feel you can't lose weight on a reduced-calorie diet, it's best to keep a detailed food diary and weigh all items except salads and vegetables for one to two weeks, then check your weight again. However, as we've said, weight loss may be slower than average if you are, say, older, or very short (see Question 1).

If you check and still find you're not losing weight, I would suggest visiting your dietician or GP for further help. Perhaps you are already at an optimum weight, or perhaps you are one of the few people with a medically recognised condition which has altered your metabolism. Indeed, some prescribed drugs, – steroids for example – can make slimming hard and weight gain easy.

8. I never used to have a weight problem, but at 40 I find I'm piling on the pounds. Is middle-aged spread inevitable?

It isn't inevitable, but it is now generally recognised that a weight gain of up to a stone from the weight of one's youthful slimness is quite acceptable, and may indeed be more healthy than trying to stay too thin as we get older.

Over the age of 30 or so, our metabolic rate (the rate at which our bodies burn up calories) begins to slow down. It is estimated that on average, for every five years over 30 we are, we need to eat 50 calories a day less than we did in our twenties in order to maintain the same weight. In other words, if you are 40, you need 100 calories a day less than you did at 30; if you are 50, you need 200 less.

This is mainly due to loss of muscle mass (it has been discovered that a man aged 75 will have less than half the muscle mass of a man in his twenties). Muscle tissue is metabolically active whereas fat tissue isn't. So with the decline in the muscle mass comes a decline in metabolic activity and a reduced need for calories.

So if you continue to eat the same as you did when you were younger – and take no extra exercise – then you can expect a small weight increase over the years. For women, this increase is not harmful, as trying to maintain too low a weight in middle age has been linked with poor bone density and increased likelihood of osteoporosis in later life, and may also predispose to a more difficult time through menopause – particularly if a diet low in essential fats (found in nuts, seeds, plant oils and fish, for example) has been followed. Many typical very low-fat slimming diets are low in these essential fats and may not be a good idea for women to follow. Essential fats – and some fat on the body – are thought to be 'nature's HRT'.

So when assessing whether your weight gain as you head towards middle age is something you should be happy about, or something to consider losing, it is best to use your common sense. If the weight is being added slowly and your Body Mass Index (see Chapter 1) is still within the acceptable range, then there is no cause for concern. But if you are piling on weight at a more alarming rate and your BMI is heading towards 30, it is unlikely that such a gain is all due to the slight lowering of metabolic rate, and more likely that you are simply eating too much and not exercising enough. A slimming programme to get your BMI down to 25–26 would then be in order.

9. Does overweight run in families?

It seems that in a reasonable percentage of cases, it does. Some scientific research has put this percentage as low as 10, other work has come up with a figure nearer 60 per cent. Whichever is correct, there is little doubt that genetic factors can predispose you to putting on weight more easily than another person. But these genetic tendencies will only cause obesity if lifestyle factors, such as the amount you eat and the amount you exercise, aren't controlled.

In other words, you may have a family tendency to put on weight – but if you eat sensibly and take enough exercise, there is no need to get hugely fat. You may, however, have to be content with being a more rounded size and shape than some of your friends. Genetic factors also control your basic body shape and where the fat is laid down. So if you are a classic 'pear', you can't turn yourself into an 'apple', for example. You can simply make the best of what you've got.

10. Why does the weight come back on again so easily at the end of a diet?

Short term, there are two major factors involved. One is psychological and possibly also physical. This is the 'yippee factor'. You reach 'the end' of your diet having, hopefully, reached target weight, and you go 'Yippee! No more boring diet food. I can eat what I like again now!' Which you do. And of course you put on weight again. If you happen to have lost a lot of weight, your normal metabolic rate will now be lower than it was when you were fat. (Remember, a 12-stone person has a higher metabolic rate than when down to 10 stone. It will **NOT** be lower than another 10-stone person of the same age and activity levels who has never dieted.)

But if you go back to eating as many calories as you did before your diet, you will get fat again. You need to eat for your new weight and new metabolism. If you have aimed for a reasonable weight, not a too-thin one, you will still be able to eat plenty.

The physical side of the 'yippee factor' may be that your body is crying out for the sustenance of which it has been deprived for a long time. This could be a consequence of a diet too low in calories or a diet too restricted in what foods you could eat.

So the motto is to slim sensibly on a varied and healthy programme including foods you enjoy, not to aim for too low a weight, and to follow a sensible interim maintenance programme such as that in Chapter 10 in the weeks after the diet has finished.

The second short-term factor is the glycogen factor. I explained on page 18 that when you start a slimming programme you will lose a few pounds of body fluids and glycogen, because of the reduction in calories and carbohydrate in your diet.

If you finish a diet on, say, 1,250 calories, and go straight back to eating 2,000 calories or so a day, then the glycogen factor will cause a weight gain, this time of a few pounds over a week or two. This won't be fat – your fat has stayed off – but it may look and feel like fat to you.

The secret of minimising the effect of the glycogen gain is gradually to build up your calorie level after you have reached your target weight. Chapter 10 shows you how to do that, so that in the few weeks after your six-week programme has finished, you will lose a little more body fat while you regain the glycogen.

Long term, there are two factors involved. The first is your lifestyle. As I said in Chapter 1, it may be easier to keep weight off by making a few pertinent lifestyle changes than by trying to fit a healthy diet into an unhealthy lifestyle. The reason many people eventually put back weight they have lost is not because their metabolic rate is shattered or that dieting has made them fat (what a preposterous idea!), but because they find it too hard within their long-term everyday life to keep up the good habits they have learnt. The factors that we discussed in Chapter 1 about just how that surplus weight accumulated are still around, and you need to remain aware of them. You need to want to be slim more than you want to eat too many calories. You need to recognise all the reasons you were overeating and make a habit of dealing with them. Chapter 10 deals with all these factors and provides tried and tested advice.

The second long-term factor is exercise. Research shows that the people with the best chance of keeping surplus weight off for good are those who exercise regularly. We explain more about this in Chapters 9 and 10.

Believe me, if you follow the advice in this book you can maintain a reasonable weight for the rest of your life. Dieting does **NOT** make you fat. You just need to get your head right.

the detox and energise plan

Often when you decide you want to lose weight, you also embark on a fitness regime – because you want not only to look better but also to feel better. It makes sense, then, to use this time when your motivation levels are so high to treat yourself to a diet that will not only help you lose pounds, but also help you to feel more energised, more healthy.

That is the basis of my Detox and Energise programme.

Detoxing

I used to think that there was no such thing as the detox effect and that products and diets claiming to help you to detox were just a con. However, having done a lot of research on the subject, I have come to the conclusion that a carefully thought-out programme can, indeed, both detox your system, re-educate your palate and re-energise your body.

To detox means to rid your body of toxins (poisons). The first questions I set out to answer were – do our bodies really carry toxins? If so, do we need help in getting rid of these? And can diet possibly do such a thing?

The answers to these three questions seem to be Yes, usually; Yes, usually; and Yes, it can.

The human body can contain toxins which have arrived in various ways: in our food and drink (pesticide and herbicide residues, hormone and antibiotic residues, artificial additives of many kinds, and alcohol, for example); because of a modern lifestyle (high levels of toxic chemicals such as carbon monoxide in the atmosphere or aluminium in pans or chemicals in food wrap, and tobacco smoke, for example); because of illness or perceived illness (viruses and bacteria are toxins, and even the 'cures' may be toxic if taken over long periods, including vitamin and mineral supplements, paracetamol and similar remedies).

If you are young, fit, healthy and stress free, your body's own defence and filter system (the lymph glands, liver and kidneys) may be able to deal with these toxins on their own, helping to remove them from the body in waste matter, urine, sweat and on the breath. But frequent ailments, feeling less than wonderful, perhaps with bloating and mildly enlarged glands around the body (the neck is a typical site for enlarged glands), all indicate that your body's toxin disposal system may need some help.

This can be done simply in three ways:

- by choosing a diet as low in probable sources of toxins as possible;
- by choosing foods, drinks and supplements which will actively aid the elimination of toxins; and
- by suitable exercise and a healthy lifestyle.

A guide to low-toxin foods and toxin-eliminating foods appears below. The diet should be followed in conjunction with the exercise tips in Chapter 9 and the lifestyle tips on page 28.

Energising

A detox regime marries very well with a revitalising, energising diet. Foods that may help your energy levels are fruits (high in natural sugars, vitamin C and phytochemicals – the 'active X factor' ingredients in natural foods that experts are now beginning to realise may hold an important key to good health and long life); vegetables (also high in vitamin C and phytochemicals as well as important minerals such as iron, selenium and calcium); complex carbohydrates (found in starchy foods such as rice and other grains, and potatoes), and essential fats (found in large quantities in plant, seed and nut oils, seeds and nuts and oily fish).

A diet combining all these foods will also be high in the anti-oxidants vitamins A, C and E and selenium. Anti-oxidants help to neutralise 'free radicals' in the body – substances which are produced in the body as a normal by-product of metabolism, but which may be produced in excess when the body is under stress or subject to pollution. It is thought that these free radicals are responsible for the human ageing process and in excess may be linked with all kinds of illnesses including cancers and arterial disease.

Weight loss

Because the Detox and Energise Plan is so natural and so naturally low in saturated fats and added sugars, most people will find that they lose weight very easily on it. There is also virtually no measuring of food which is another bonus.

How the plan works

Lots of detox programmes last for only two or three days and throw you straight in at the deep end – going directly from your normal eating habits to a virtual fast. A short, sharp detox like that isn't ideal.

For one thing it is always best to prepare your body – and your mind – for a detox programme by going into it gradually. Your digestive system needs to adjust over a period of a week or two otherwise you could suffer from indigestion, wind and perhaps a loose bowel. And for another thing, it takes more than a couple of days for the detoxification to work. Toxins that the lymph, liver and kidneys have not been able to deal with are stored in body fat and, as we've seen, you can't lose more than a tiny amount of body fat in a day or two.

Lastly, a fast or near-fast will nearly always result in your feeling lethargic and perhaps dizzy with a headache and will also result in unnecessary loss of lean body tissue from muscle and organs.

There is no need to fast in order to detox. My gradual plan helps to eliminate these symptoms and should actually help to energise you.

What you are going to do, then, is gradually to cut down – or in some cases cut out – the dietary items that may have been contributing to a toxic state, while gradually building up the 'good' items. Think of the six weeks as a 'U curve' with weeks three and four the base of the curve when your detox regime will be at its most 'pure', consisting of almost nothing but plant foods. The whole thing is a fairly gentle process but by the end of the six weeks you should feel wonderful!

Exercise

For the detox to work at optimum level, you need to take regular moderate exercise outdoors. This is to help stimulate your lymph glands to work efficiently and is particularly important if you have been prone to fluid retention and bloating. Have you ever noticed how you need to 'go to the loo' when you come in from a brisk walk, cycle ride, swim or whatever? That is because the exercise has stimulated the lymph system. Your blood flow is also improved which helps in the detox process. You will have 'worked up a sweat', eliminating toxins that way. And lastly you should have filled your lungs with oxygen-rich air, helping to remove toxins through the breath. All in all – exercise is vital and re-vitalising! Read Chapter 9 for all the information you need.

Lifestyle

As I have said, some toxins are present because of a poor lifestyle. While following the Detox and Energise Plan, you should not smoke tobacco, drink alcohol or take drugs of any kind other than mandatory ones prescribed by your doctor. (If you have any particular medical conditions you should ask your doctor if this plan is suitable for you to follow.) You should also avoid vitamin and mineral supplements unless completely natural (lots of supplements are artificially manufactured and may themselves contain possible toxins or allergens).

You should get plenty of sleep, rest and relaxation and try to reduce stress levels. You should sleep with an open window in a cool room. And you should make time for yourself and your diet.

Organic food

Ideally you should eat and drink nothing but organic produce while on the detox. This will be guaranteed free from agro-chemicals and additives. All of our basic food – fruit, vegetables, milk, flesh, eggs and so on – may contain traces of residues such as pesticides, herbicides and fungicides.

All major supermarkets now have a wide range of organic produce on offer. You can also join a box scheme, where organic produce is delivered to your door weekly (for information telephone the Soil Association on 0117 929 0661). You can also look in the small ad columns of Sunday papers, food magazines and so on for small companies who specialise in various types of organic produce by mail order – these are particularly good for meat, fish and cheese. Yes, organic food does cost up to 30 per cent more than mass-produced non-organic food, but I have found that most people beginning a plan such as this one will actually find that they save money on their grocery bill over the six weeks. That is because 'added value' high-cost foods – processed, ready to eat, take-aways, and so on – are not featured, and also because the overall calorie consumption is reduced. What you save on all the junk and unnecessary food you spend on gorgeous, wholesome, better-tasting food that really is good for you! Don't begrudge it.

Here is a list of items that you should seek out in their organic form:

- Poultry
- Fish
- Eggs
- Dairy produce
- Fruit
- Vegetables
- Pulses
- Bread
- Grains, including rice, breakfast cereals, etc.

Wholefoods

During the programme, all your foods should be 'whole' – in other words, not refined. Avoid white bread, white rice, white pasta, refined sugar, anything other than whole-grain breakfast cereals and so on. Wholefoods contain more vital vitamins such as the B-group, more fibre for a healthy digestive system and more of some other trace elements.

Pulses can be canned in water, but not in brine. Rinse and drain well before use.

Where to obtain the more unusual detox plants, herbs, etc.

You will find some fairly unusual plants, herbs, roots, etc. listed below, all of which can help your body to eliminate toxins. You will not find many of them in your local supermarket and you may need either to visit a well-stocked health-food shop which should keep organic dried versions of the items mentioned, or else send off for a mail order catalogue to a reputable company, such as Neal's Yard Remedies (telephone 0161 831 7875 for details).

If you live in the country, you may also be able to pick some of the plants yourself – even from your own garden! Who hasn't got dandelion and nettles growing somewhere near by, for example? If you are going to try seeking some of the other plants, arm yourself with a good book on wild food (such as Richard Mabey's **FOOD FOR FREE**) so that you don't end up picking the wrong thing and poisoning yourself – **NOT** the idea of this plan at all! Wash all plants thoroughly and avoid using plants that have been growing close to a road. Page 42 explains how to make your own herbal teas and decoctions. It is very easy.

Getting organised

Before you begin, sort out your store-cupboard, refrigerator, etc., and chuck out things that you won't want to be eating, to make room for the items that you will.

Make a shopping list to take you through at least the first week, and thereafter shop regularly for what you need.

Store your food in cool and dark conditions, properly wrapped, to retain maximum vitamins C and B, and use it regularly.

Because you will be 'de-cluttering' your eating life (this plan is ideal for minimalists) you should in the long run save time on your food.

Foods and drinks to help your detox

These pages are a quick reference to good sources of a variety of nutrients and plant chemicals which will aid your Detox and Energise Plan. Over the weeks ahead they will come to form a large part of your diet. Consult the six-week plan for their usage.

- *Vitamin C*   A powerful anti-oxidant which helps maintain healthy skin, gums, eyes. Also important for absorption of iron. Excellent sources – blackcurrants, kiwi fruit, rose hips, citrus fruits, sweet peppers, broccoli, sprouts, parsley, strawberries, mango, guava, melon, tomatoes, leafy greens, fresh chilli peppers. Most fresh and frozen fruits and vegetables contain some vitamin C; canned contain very little and should be avoided. Storage, light and heat deplete foods of their vitamin C content.
- *Vitamin E*   Another anti-oxidant vital for healthy soft skin, its anti-ageing properties, and its ability to bolster the body's immune system. Excellent sources – wheatgerm oil, sunflower oil and seeds, safflower oil, hazelnuts, sun-dried tomatoes,

almonds, corn oil, groundnut oil, pine nuts, Brazil nuts, sweet potato, other nuts.* Store E-rich oily foods in cool dark conditions and use quickly – they can go rancid and oxidise.

- **Vitamin B group** Six individual vitamins that work together to help the body maintain metabolic processes, energy levels and in various other tasks. Good sources – whole grains, fish, eggs, poultry, lean pork, yeast extract, but also present in a wide variety of healthy foods and so a varied diet is essential.

- **Beta-carotene** Anti-oxidant which helps boost the immune system and mop up surplus free radicals. Excellent sources – carrots, sweet potato, dark leafy greens, sweet peppers, chilli peppers, orange-fleshed squash, orange-fleshed melon, mango, tomatoes, broccoli.

- **Selenium** Anti-oxidant mineral which works with vitamin E. Strong likelihood of shortage in the diet. Excellent sources – Brazil nuts. Good sources – green or brown lentils, canned or fresh tuna, mullet, squid, sardines, sunflower seeds, white fish, wholemeal bread, salmon, walnuts, lean pork.

- **Zinc** Another anti-oxidant mineral important to help keep the liver healthy and eliminate toxins. Good sources – wheatgerm, seeds, nuts, All-Bran, shellfish, lean red meat, Quorn.

- **Iron** Carries oxygen from the lungs through the body, helps healing and the immune system. Lack of iron (fairly common in females) can cause lethargy and lack of energy. Excellent low saturated-fat sources of iron – ground ginger, seaweed, All-Bran, green or brown lentils, sesame and pumpkin seeds, soya beans, Weetabix, dried peaches and apricots, bulghar wheat, pot barley, brown rice, dark leafy greens, broccoli. Lean red meat and eggs are a good source of easily absorbed iron and are allowed in the first two weeks of the diet but contain a moderate amount of saturated fat.

- **Essential fats** Two types of polyunsaturated fat which are important for the smooth and efficient functioning of the body including weight control. May also help the immune system and to maintain energy levels. Essential fats are found in excellent quantities in seed and nut oils as well as in seeds and nuts themselves. Several other plant foods and fish contain reasonable amounts of one or other of the two essential fatty acids.

- **Fibre** Adequate fibre in the diet is important on this plan to help the speedy passage of food through the gut thus helping the elimination process. It will also help prevent hunger. Fibre is found only in plant foods. Excellent sources are pulses, pot barley, All-Bran, whole grains, peas and beans, parsnips, sprouts, dried apricots, figs and prunes, leafy green vegetables. All unrefined plant foods contain some fibre. Refined cereals contain very little.

- **Diuretics** Certain plants can help the body eliminate fluid in the urine quickly – important if you are prone to fluid retention and bloating. Some of these are dandelion, nettles, parsley, tarragon, dock root, cucumber, onions and apples.

- **Plants to aid liver function** Poor liver and gallbladder function can slow down the elimination of toxins. Help your liver cope with the aid of dandelion root, marigold, parsley, burdock leaves or root, peppermint leaves, dock root, apples, cucumber, onions, artichoke hearts, beetroot juice and olive oil. A supplement of milk thistle can also be taken, available from health food shops or by mail order.

- **Plants to aid lymph function** Stimulate your lymph system into working well with the help of angelica, lovage, marigold, rosemary, dock, ginger, cayenne, oregano.

- **Laxatives** Natural laxatives can be incorporated into the diet to help eliminate waste matter. These are rhubarb, prunes, licorice, olive oil, burdock,

* ALL NUTS MUST BE FRESH, NOT SALTED.

dock, and aloe vera juice. All the high-fibre foods will also help to prevent constipation.

- *Heating foods* Elimination through perspiration can be increased by including 'heating' foods in the diet. These are most spices, particularly mustard and chillies; garlic, onions, green tea, rosemary and thyme.

(See page 42 for details of how to make your own herbal drinks. See the six-week programme for suggestions on using herbs within the diet.)

What to do

All you do is check out the the list on pages 29–31 which details all the 'detox' foods and drinks that you should have plenty of over the six-week programme, and the reasons why. See below a list of 'unlimited' foods/drink that you can have freely throughout the six weeks.

Then follow the plan which is a 'page to a week' for the next six weeks. Every day you will choose a Breakfast, a Lunch, an Evening Meal and two Snacks plus at least four pints of liquid a day. (Unless stated, all portion sizes of fruits, vegetables and salads are large, and all portions of any other foods are

medium.) You can choose from the meals suggested or decide on your own meals as long as they are in line with the 'goals for the week' listing foods to avoid, foods to eat more of and foods to go easy on at the start of each week's page.

After the six weeks is up, you will then find a page on what to do when the detox is over. This advice is more specific to you than the more general advice you will find in Chapter 10.

Unlimiteds

- *Foods* All organic fresh and frozen green vegetables and salad items.
- *Condiments* Fresh herbs or dried herbs and spices, lemon juice, unsalted tomato purée, passata, good quality wine vinegar, unsalted vegetable stock/cubes.
- *Drinks* Water, mineral water, organic herbal teas, decoctions and concoctions (see page 42); unsweetened fruit teas, green tea; fresh home-made fruit juices diluted with water; fresh home-made vegetable juices. (**NOTE** limit carrot juice to one glass a day).

Remember to drink four pints of fluid a day.

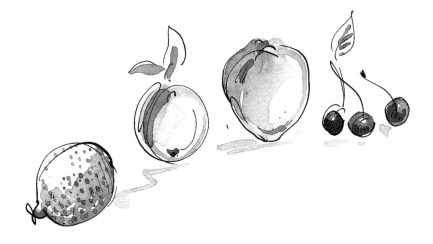

WEEK ONE

Goals for the week

Eat/drink more

- Fresh fruits, especially any of those listed on pages 29–30 which are rich in vitamin C or beta-carotene, or apples. Aim for three portions a day. This is easy to do if you have fruit every day at breakfast, with/as one snack a day and at either lunchtime or after your evening meal.
- Leafy green vegetables. Aim for a minimum of one portion a day.
- Water or similar. Four pints a day is ideal. Herbal teas count towards your water intake. This week try dandelion-root tea to help liver function (see recipe page 42) or try any of the herbs mentioned in the list on page 30.

Cut down on

- Added salt. Stop adding salt to food on your plate and cut down on the amount you add in cooking.
- Fat. Choose lean meats and give yourself smaller portions than usual, remove all visible fat off food, cut by half the fat you put on bread, etc., skim all fat off pan juices when roasting before making gravy/sauce, and try to choose lower-fat cheeses such as Brie, Camembert, Edam, feta, light cream cheese, half-fat Cheddar, Halloumi and cottage cheese rather than higher-fat ones like Cheddar, Stilton, cream cheese and Cambazola.
- Caffeine. Cut down on the amount of tea and/or coffee that you drink. Make it weaker. (Choose herbal drinks instead, see below and page 42.) Cut down on the amount of chocolate you eat and choose good quality plain organic chocolate (e.g. Green and Black).

- Highly processed foods. Try to avoid packet and canned foods, especially those with lots of E numbers (read the ingredients label), such as soups, sauce mixes, snack foods, instant desserts.

Avoid

- Added sugar. Don't add sugar to cereals, drinks, etc. Try to do without artificial sweetener. If necessary, cut down the amount of sugar you use gradually this week, day by day.
- Sweet, highly refined foods. Avoid cakes, packet biscuits, sugary desserts, sweet pastries, baked goods and all confectionery except good chocolate.
- All pastry.
- Take-away meals and ready to heat meals.
- Cola and all other carbonated commercial drinks.
- Percolated coffee and cafetière coffee.
- All milk except skimmed milk or soya milk.

Notes

- Don't forget your unlimited items listed on page 31.
- Have a Breakfast, Lunch, Evening Meal plus two healthy Snacks and plenty to drink every day. Do try to make your own fresh fruit and vegetable juices. Any juices mentioned in the meal suggestions are ideas only – feel free to juice whenever you like.
- Try to buy everything organic, or at least free range.
- Eat enough to satisfy hunger but no more.
- Each week the meal suggestions are samples only; try to add a few ideas of your own that fit in with the guidelines above and include plenty of unlimited items.

Breakfasts

- Portion vitamin C- and/or fibre-rich fruit; All-Bran; natural bio yogurt.
- Brown toast with a scraping of butter; low-sugar jam; natural bio yogurt; fresh citrus juice.
- 'No added sugar or salt' muesli, with 1 banana and skimmed milk to cover.
- Boiled egg; 1 slice wholewheat toast with a scraping of butter; 1 portion vitamin C and/or fibre-rich fruit.

Lunches

- Wholewheat sandwich filled with Brie and sliced tomato; 1 portion fruit of choice; 1 slice malt loaf.
- Low-salt baked beans on toast; vitamin C-rich fruit; 1 apple.
- Lean cooked chicken with tomato, green pepper and Cos salad; Ryvitas; 1 fruit-flavoured fromage frais; 1 portion fruit of choice.
- Eggs on brown toast with a scraping of butter; 1 orange; 1 Greek yogurt.
- Wholewheat pasta, avocado and tomato salad; 1 small portion grilled Halloumi cheese; beetroot or apple juice.

Evening Meals

- Small lean steak; new potatoes; leafy greens; peas; apricot juice.
- Baked white fish; oven chips; peas; tomato salad.
- Brown rice topped with selection of grilled Mediterranean vegetables and garnished with either small amount of grated Parmesan cheese or poached egg; fresh fruit juice.
- Baked potato; baked beans *or* home-made chilli con carne; large mixed salad.
- Roast or grilled chicken or turkey (skin removed) with lemon and tarragon; new potatoes; broccoli; puréed parsnips; carrots; skimmed pan juices.

Snacks

- Fresh fruit.
- Staffordshire oatcake and hummus.
- Small piece plain organic chocolate or cheese and apple.
- Bio yogurt with fruit purée.

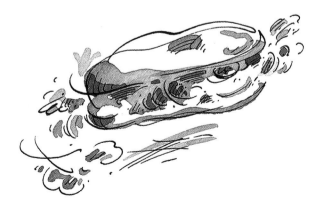

WEEK TWO

Goals for the week

Eat more

All items as Week 1 plus:
- Salad, including tomatoes, onions, cucumber, dark lettuce leaves, rocket, watercress, spinach.
- Fresh herbs – see page 29.
- Fish, both white and oily. Mackerel, herring, salmon, trout, sardines and tuna are oily.
- Dried fruits – go for apricots, peaches, prunes and figs rather than sultanas, raisins and currants.

Try to cut down on

- High salt foods. These include many cheeses, processed foods, soy sauce.
- Added salt. Cut again the amount you use in cooking.
- Chocolate. Cut down again on the amount of chocolate you eat; limit to one square a day.
- All animal flesh. Limit to twice in the week.
- Bread and wheat-based products such as crackers. Limit bread to one slice a day.

Avoid

All items as Week 1 plus:
- Refined flour, cereals and grains. That includes all bread except wholemeal, breakfast cereals such as cornflakes, crisped rice, white pasta, white rice.
- All highly processed packet foods and all canned foods except pulses canned in water and tomatoes.
- Black tea, coffee, squashes.
- Full-fat cheese, including Cheddar, Stilton, soft blue cheeses, cream cheese.

Notes

As Week 1.

Breakfasts

- Fresh berry fruits; natural low-fat bio yogurt; oat flakes.
- Fruit Compôte (see recipe page 43); natural 8 per cent fat fromage frais; muesli; fresh fruit juice.
- Fresh citrus fruit salad; Greek yogurt; grapenuts.
- Boiled egg; 2 rye crispbreads or 1 small slice whole rye bread; 1 orange.

Lunches

- Tabbouleh (see recipe page 42); 1 apple; 1 low-fat bio yogurt; beetroot juice.
- Brown rice and tuna (canned in water, drained) salad with watercress, hard-boiled egg, spinach and parsley; citrus juice.
- Salad of new potatoes with chopped mint, parsley, broad beans tossed in bio yogurt and lemon juice dressing; green salad; dried apricots.
- Salad of brown rice, chopped apple, chopped dried apricot, a little lean chicken; herb salad.
- Broccoli, Potato and Garlic Soup (see recipe page 42), ½ slice wholemeal bread; large mixed salad; 1 banana.

Evening Meals

- Poached salmon; new potatoes; large mixed salad or broccoli and peas.
- Lean chicken or turkey stir-fried in groundnut oil with selection of fresh vegetables; 1 small portion wholewheat noodles; Fruit Compôte (see recipe page 43)
- Sweet Potato Curry (see recipe page 43) and brown rice; portion vitamin C-rich fruit.
- White fish, grilled or baked; lemon; peas; green beans.
- Baked potato; natural 8 per cent fromage frais mixed with mustard; large mixed salad.

Snacks

- Rye crispbread and hummus.
- Fresh fruit.
- Dried fruit.
- Low-fat bio yogurt and apple.

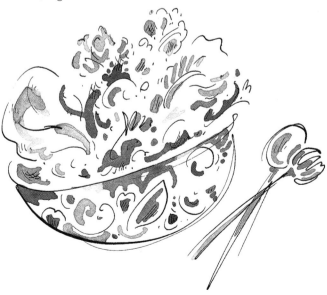

WEEK THREE

Goals for the week

Eat more

All items as previous weeks plus:
- Olive oil and other plant oils high in essential fatty acids.
- Fresh juices. Squeeze your own citrus juices. If you have a blender you can whizz all kinds of fruits and vegetables to make a 'complete' juice including the fruit/vegetable fibre. Juice extractors leave much of the fruit's goodness behind in the pulp.
- Herbal teas and herbs. The herbs listed on page 30 really do have a beneficial effect in helping your body to 'detox' – give some of them a try. One to two cups a day should help. Add fresh herbs to salads and sprinkle over vegetables. Garlic is another good herb to use regularly.
- Pulses. Now you've cut out meat, replace it in your diet with more high-protein, low-fat pulses such as kidney beans, soya beans (and tofu, which is made from soya), butter beans, chickpeas and lentils. They can be mixed into salads, served as a vegetable or used to replace meat in dishes such as curries and casseroles.
- Raw foods. Eat more salads and nibble on raw vegetables during the day. Uncooked vegetables retain more of their vitamin C and can seem more filling.

Cut down on

- Grains of all kinds including breakfast cereals, rice, bulghar.
- Starchy vegetables such as potatoes, parsnips, sweetcorn, beetroot – have small portions only.

Avoid

All items as previous weeks plus:
- All bread and wheat products.
- Added salt – your tastebuds should have acclimatised by now.
- Chocolate.
- All dairy produce except skimmed milk and natural low-fat bio yogurt.
- Eggs.
- All meat, poultry and game.

Notes

As Week 1 plus:
- Calcium – It is important to get adequate calcium in the diet. One of our main sources is hard cheese and other dairy produce. As you are cutting right down on dairy products now it is vital to get calcium from other sources. Eat plenty of seeds, tofu, almonds, figs, Brazil nuts, dark green leafy vegetables and broccoli as well as unlimited low-fat bio yogurt and ½ pint of skimmed milk or calcium-fortified soya milk daily. Milk can be blended with fruit for a morning shake.

Breakfasts

- Every day have a selection of fresh fruit and dried fruit with plenty of low-fat bio yogurt and a small handful of 'no added sugar or salt' muesli, plus a juice. Sprinkle with wheatgerm if liked.

Lunches

- Large fresh mixed salad including fresh herbs such as parsley and dark leaves such as rocket, spinach, lamb's lettuce; olive oil and vinegar dressing; small portion hummus made by blending cooked chickpeas with olive oil, lemon juice and black pepper; beetroot juice.
- Large fresh salad as above; sliced avocado and pine nuts mixed with 2 tablespoons cooked brown rice; apple juice.
- Fresh carrot and tomato soup (from chilled counter or home made); chopped parsley; fruit.
- Purée of butter beans (blended with a little olive oil and lemon juice) with selection of raw crudités; fruit.
- Broccoli soup (made by cooking broccoli in vegetable stock and puréeing); 1 banana.

Evening Meals

- Small baked potato; selection of steamed or baked Mediterranean vegetables including red peppers, onions, drizzled with olive or groundnut oil; peach juice.
- Stir-fried vegetables in sesame oil with cubed tofu, beansprouts, cabbage; carrots or similar; nuts or seeds; 1 slice melon.
- 2 tablespoons cooked brown rice with Aubergine and Lentil Curry (see recipe page 111); 1 tablespoon low-fat bio yogurt; 1 orange.
- Baked trout with handful almonds; broccoli; spinach; fruit.
- Large mixed salad with olive oil dressing; sunflower seeds; 1 banana.

Snacks

- Fruit.
- Dried fruit.
- Bio yogurt.
- Avocado purée with crudités.
- Skimmed milk and fruit blended into a shake with a little wheatgerm or wheatgerm oil if liked.

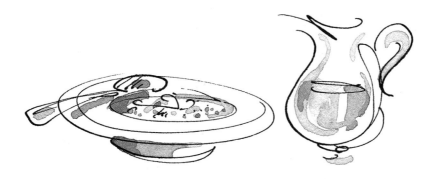

WEEK FOUR

Goals for the week

Eat more

As previous weeks, with the exception of pulses and dried fruits, plus:

- Nuts and seeds. These are full of essential fatty acids as well as protein, and contain calcium.
- Beansprouts. Contain vitamin C as well as protein.
- Raw foods.

Cut down on

- Pulses. This is a very light calorie week.
- Dried fruits (same reason).

Avoid

As previous weeks plus:
- All starchy vegetables, all grains, fish.

Notes
As Week 1 plus:

- To drink – remember to have plenty of water during the days, as well as herbal teas, green tea and diluted fruit and vegetable juices.
- Yogurt can be substituted with calcium-fortified soya yogurt if you prefer.
- Try to take it easy this week, which is the peak of your detox diet. You shouldn't feel hungry but if you do, have plenty of snacks during the day from the unlimited lists or the snack suggestions below.
- Remember to get plenty of calcium-rich foods (see list Week 3) and a twice-daily herbal infusion – try dandelion and burdock plus nettle.
- Substitute dairy skimmed milk and low-fat yogurt with calcium-enriched soya milk and yogurt.

Breakfasts

- Fresh fruit and calcium-enriched soya yogurt with chopped walnuts, Brazil nuts, almonds and sunflower seeds, wheatgerm; fresh fruit juice.

Lunches

- Beansprout, beetroot and carrot salad with hazelnuts and pine nuts, tossed in olive oil and lemon juice dressing; fresh fruit plus fruit juice.
- Salad of avocado, tomato and onion; fruit and pumpkin seeds.
- Handful Brazil nuts; large green and herb salad; fresh vegetable juice.
- Coleslaw made with shredded cabbage, carrot and onion, chopped apple, walnut pieces and pine nuts tossed in lemon juice and calcium-enriched soya yogurt dressing; fruit juice.

Evening Meals

- Stir-fry of a little Quorn with beansprouts, fresh cashew nuts, selection of vegetables; fruit.
- Aubergine chips brushed with olive oil and baked until tender; calcium-enriched soya yogurt, garlic and cucumber dip; green salad; fruit and seeds.
- Lentil purée dip; crudités; fruit and seeds.
- Green salad topped with slices of avocado and grilled red pepper strips; handful Brazil nuts; fruit.

Snacks

- Crudités with avocado dip.
- Fruit.
- Sunflower or other seeds.
- Calcium-enriched soya yogurt.

WEEK FIVE

Goals for the week

Eat more

- Small portions starchy vegetables can be included in the diet again this week.
- Pulses can be eaten in larger portions again.
- Skimmed milk, low-fat fromage frais and Quorn can be included again this week. Calcium-enriched soya products can be used instead of milk and yogurt again if liked.
- Fish can be added to the diet as well.
- The rest of the programme is the same as Week 4.

Notes

As Week 1 plus:

- In the last two weeks of the programme you can gradually add more foods to your diet. If you notice any bad reaction to a food (bloating, wind, for example) it may be that you are intolerant of that food. Cut it out again and ask your GP to refer you to a dietician for further advice.

Breakfasts

- Shake of skimmed milk blended with banana and berries and topped with wheatgerm.
- Bio yogurt with Fruit Compôte (see recipe page 43) and sunflower seeds.
- Bio yogurt with fresh fruit, mixed nuts and pumpkin seeds.

Lunches

- Large mixed salad with olive oil dressing and raw mushrooms marinated in red wine vinegar, herbs and groundnut oil overnight.
- Cooked Puy lentils tossed in olive oil and lemon dressing; large green and herb salad.
- Fresh chilled or home-made tomato and basil soup with fromage frais drizzled in; fruit.
- Small portion tuna in water, drained; tomato and onion salad; 1 banana.
- Hummus (see page 37) with crudités; 1 apple; 1 bio yogurt.

Evening Meals

- Vegetable and tofu stir-fry as Week 3.
- Lentil and potato soup (made by simmering green lentils and diced potato in vegetable stock, then puréeing); 1 banana.
- Small steak of fresh tuna, pan-fried in groundnut oil; small portion new potatoes; green beans; broccoli; fruit juice.
- Casserole of Quorn with potatoes, mushrooms, canned tomatoes, fresh herbs.
- Grilled sardines; large mixed salad with olive oil dressing; 1 apple.

Snacks

- Lentil purée dip and crudités.
- Fruit.
- Almonds.

WEEK SIX

Goals for the week

Add to your diet this week

- Whole grains (see note below first) including bread, cereals.
- Dried fruit.
- Eggs.
- Lean meat, poultry and game if liked.
- Whole-milk bio yogurt.
- A little butter and honey can be added to the diet if liked.
- Rest of diet as Week 5.

Notes

As Week 1 plus:
- If you add cereals, grains and bread to your diet and experience a reaction such as bloating, wind, you may be intolerant. Try omitting wheat products from the diet for a further week and if symptoms subside you may have a wheat intolerance. (Wheatgerm or wheatgerm oil are unlikely to produce a reaction.) If symptoms persist, you may be intolerant to other grains, such as rye or oats. See your GP and ask for an appointment with the dietician for further advice.

Breakfasts

- Muesli with chopped walnuts added, skimmed milk to cover and 1 banana; fruit juice.
- Shredded Wheat with skimmed milk to cover, with strawberries, poppy seeds.
- Whole-milk yogurt; muesli; 1 apple; sunflower seeds.

- Rye bread, butter, pure fruit spread, orange, low-fat bio yogurt, handful Brazil nuts.
- Whole-milk bio yogurt, honey; Fruit Compôte (see recipe page 43); wheatgerm.

Lunches

- Poached egg; rye bread; large mixed salad.
- Cooked brown rice tossed with a little lean cooked chopped chicken, orange slices and walnuts with olive oil and orange juice dressing.
- Cold fresh poached salmon and cold wholewheat cooked pasta shapes tossed with home-made pesto sauce (no Parmesan); green salad.
- Broccoli, Potato and Garlic Soup (see recipe page 42); rye bread; fruit.
- Turkey and salad sandwich on wholemeal bread; 1 banana.
- Wholewheat pitta filled with hummus and salad; 1 orange.

Evening Meals

- Flat Mushrooms Stuffed with Pine Nut Risotto (see recipe page 108); mixed salad; almonds; 1 apple.
- Small portion baked chicken with garlic and lemon; sweet potato; broccoli; peas.
- Home-made Ratatouille (see recipe page 111) topped with poached egg on bed of bulghar wheat.
- Swordfish and Red Pepper Kebabs (see recipe page 60); Tabbouleh (see recipe page 42); dried apricots; Brazil nuts.
- Medallions of pork fillet pan-fried in olive oil with slices of apple; new potatoes; spring greens; green beans.

Snacks

- Sunflower or other seeds.
- Fruit.
- Hummus and crudités.
- Almonds, Brazil nuts or walnuts.

What to do next

When you have completed your six-week Detox and Energise programme you should have lost your surplus weight and should be feeling marvellous.

Because the programme has been so gradual – slowly taking you **DOWN** to an almost pure fruit and vegetable diet, then slowly taking you **UP** again to a wide variety of foods, your tastebuds will be acclimatised to fresh, natural tastes. Your old liking for sugary, salty foods should have disappeared for good and you should find it easy from now on to eat a healthy diet, low in processed and low-nutrient foods, to maintain your new weight and to stay well and full of energy. Then your future maintenance diet will not include a return to all your old bad eating habits.

To sum up, this will be:

A diet similar to that of Week 6 but adding:

- Occasional 'treats' as you like – e.g. good quality chocolate, good quality wine (both preferably organic), home-made wholefood biscuits and cakes.
- Small amounts of high-fat dairy produce – e.g. Cheddar cheese, cream, ice cream from time to time if you like.
- Small amounts of coffee and tea.
- White bread sometimes if liked, and if it causes no adverse symptoms.

Try to avoid permanently:

- Added sugar and salt.
- Low-quality processed packet and tinned products containing lots of additives.
- High salt intake.
- Pastry, commercial cakes and baked goods, packet biscuits.
- Large amounts of high saturated-fat foods such as hard cheeses, cream and soft blue cheeses, fatty cuts of red meat, cream, eggs, butter.

And also try to:

- Continue buying organic produce whenever you can.
- Start your own vegetable and herb patch and use organic methods.
- Lead as clean, healthy and stress-free a life as you can.

To sum up, your diet will be:

- High in fresh fruits and vegetables.
- High in raw salads.
- High in essential fatty acids found in plant oils, nuts, seeds and fish.
- High in pulses.
- High in unrefined cereal foods, particularly those which don't cause a problem for you.
- High in water. (Detox infusions and decoctions should be taken in moderate quantities only and as needed.)
- It will also include lean meat, poultry, white fish (unless vegetarian) and low-fat milk, cheeses and yogurt or soya alternatives, and dried fruits.

For further tips on avoiding weight gain in the future, turn to Chapter 10.

RECIPES FOR YOUR DETOX AND ENERGISE PLAN

INFUSIONS

An infusion is simply made as you would make ordinary tea. You make it from leaves or flowers of the plant, and it can also be called a tisane. Typical herbs that you might use to make an infusion are nettles, dandelion leaves, mint, lemon balm, marigold, rosemary or thyme.

The normal quantity of herb to water is one good tablespoon of fresh herb to half a pint of water. You can also use dried leaves or flowers to make an infusion, in which case one heaped teaspoonful is about the right amount.

Simply put the fresh or dried herb in a teapot or jug, pour on boiling water and leave to infuse for 5 minutes or so. Pour the tea into your cup or mug through a tea strainer and drink.

DECOCTIONS

Sometimes you may be using a part of the plant that is too tough or woody to make a good infusion – dandelion root or cinnamon sticks are two examples. In this case you need to decoct the herb. This means you chop it up and simmer it, uncovered, for about half an hour in water until enough of the 'active ingredient' of the herb has been released and the liquid is reduced by a third to a half, then strain and drink (or cool and refrigerate until needed). For one serving, one good tablespoon of chopped fresh plant or one good teaspoonful of dried plant to 250ml of water is about right.

BROCCOLI, POTATO AND GARLIC SOUP

Serves 2
175 calories and 6g fat per portion

1 dessertspoon sunflower seed oil
1 medium onion, chopped
1 large clove garlic, peeled and crushed
150g potato, peeled and chopped small
Black pepper
400ml organic low-salt vegetable stock
100g broccoli florets
1 dessertspoon chopped fresh mint
1 dessertspoon chopped fresh parsley
Low salt substitute (optional)
2 dessertspoons natural bio yogurt

Heat the oil in a saucepan and cook the onion over a medium low heat until softened, stirring occasionally. Add the garlic, potato, pepper and stock and bring to a simmer; cook for 15 minutes. Add the broccoli and simmer for another 5–7 minutes, then purée the soup in an electric blender. Return to the pan, stir in the mint, parsley and salt substitute if using, reheat, then serve with the yogurt swirled in.

NOTE *Home-made stock is easy to make – simply simmer carrot, onion, leek, celery in water with a small bouquet garni (or a few sprigs of thyme and parsley) for 30 minutes, then strain off the liquid.*

TABBOULEH

Serves 2
160 calories and 6.5g fat per portion

50g bulghar wheat
1 Little Gem lettuce or half a head of Cos

I beef tomato, deseeded and chopped

4 spring onions, chopped

4cm chunk cucumber, chopped

I handful fresh mint, chopped

I handful fresh parsley, chopped

I tablespoon olive oil

I tablespoon lemon juice

Black pepper

Soak the bulghar wheat in just boiled water for 20 minutes and drain thoroughly. Slice the lettuce thinly lengthways and arrange on plates. In a bowl, mix together the bulghar wheat with the remaining ingredients and pile onto the lettuce.

SWEET POTATO CURRY

Serves 2
370 calories and 8g fat per portion

I tablespoon groundnut oil

I medium onion, thinly sliced

I large or 2 small sweet potatoes (about 350g), peeled and cut into cubes

I clove garlic, peeled and crushed

½ teaspoon each of ground chilli, cumin, ginger, turmeric and coriander seed

150g broccoli florets, parboiled

50g green lentils, simmered in water until tender and drained

200ml low-salt vegetable stock

100g baby leaf spinach or shredded spring greens

Black pepper

2 tablespoons natural whole-milk bio yogurt

Heat the oil in a large non-stick frying pan and sauté the onion and sweet potato over a medium high heat, stirring frequently, until part cooked and the potato is tinged golden. Add the garlic and spices and stir for a minute or two, then add the broccoli, lentils and stock, bring to a simmer, and cook, uncovered, for 10 minutes or until the sweet potato and broccoli is almost cooked. Add the spinach (or greens), black pepper and yogurt and stir, simmer for a minute to wilt the greens, then serve. This is good served with chopped cucumber tossed in a little low-fat bio yogurt plus finely chopped garlic, if liked.

NOTE *You can substitute some of the spinach or greens with fresh nettle leaves if available.*

FRUIT COMPÔTE

Serves 4
110 calories and trace fat per portion

50g dried apricots

50g dried peaches

50g stoned dried prunes

50g dried figs

300ml fresh orange juice

Cinnamon stick

2 cloves

Lemon zest

Put the dried fruits in a saucepan, cover with the orange juice, adding water to cover as necessary. Tuck in the remaining ingredients and simmer, covered, for 30 minutes or until all the fruit is tender. Remove the cinnamon stick and cloves and serve warm or allow to cool. Store in an airtight container in the refrigerator for a maximum of 3 days.

NOTE *Fresh chopped fruit and/or nuts and seeds can be added to the compôte before serving.*

CASE HISTORY

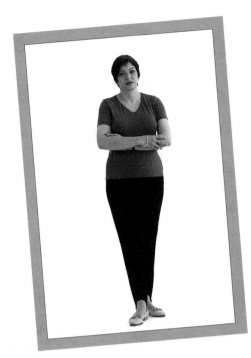

PAM LAWRENSON

AGE: **44**

STATUS: **Married; no children**

OCCUPATION: **Marketing and management consultant**

HEIGHT: **5 ft 5 ins**

START WEIGHT: **10 st 13 lb**

WEIGHT AFTER SIX WEEKS: **10 st 1 $\frac{1}{2}$ lb**

START BMI: **26.4**

BMI AFTER SIX WEEKS: **24.5**

START STATISTICS: **38–31–41**

STATISTICS AFTER SIX WEEKS: **36$\frac{1}{2}$–27$\frac{3}{4}$–39**

Pam had been slim with no real bother for most of her adult life, until about three years ago she began to put on weight. 'My husband and I have quite a full social life and I think this must have been the main reason; coupled with not exercising as much as I should have, and grabbing quick, high-fat meals when I was busy.'

When Pam contacted me she had also been made redundant from her long-term job and was in real need of a boost to her looks and confidence. 'I was flabby all over with a bloated stomach and heavy thighs. I couldn't get into a lot of my clothes and was always conscious that I didn't look good.' Pam had been trying to lose weight by herself for over six months with little or no success. 'Despite going to the gym three times a week and going for a 3-mile run once a week, I lost only half a pound, but didn't know what I was doing wrong.'

Pam's pre-plan food diary showed me that she was eating about 250 calories a day too much for her own needs; about 40 per cent of her diet was fat and she'd sometimes eat things like tuna and mayonnaise or cheese straws for breakfast! Although the exercise was probably keeping even more pounds at bay, it wasn't burning enough calories to help her lose weight – the gym work wasn't aerobic and her running not frequent enough.

Pam really wanted to change her eating habits and retune her tastebuds. 'I like the idea of the Detox plan,' she said. 'But I often have to entertain and eat out, I also like to eat in the evening with my husband who will want his normal meals, and we are going to the United States for a 10-day holiday right in the middle of the six-week programme! What can I do?'

We came to a compromise, which was that Pam would follow the Detox Plan as far as she could and at times when she couldn't, would simply switch to the meal suggestions in the Business Plan. This worked very well. Says Pam, 'During the six weeks, I/we ate out 18 times, entertained 23 people, had 10 days away in America (where they really like their food!), and I had a two-day course where the food was provided. Despite all this, I lost nearly 12 pounds, and a lot of inches, including 2 inches off each thigh, which was great.

'I was delighted to find I could still lose weight without having radically to alter my lifestyle, which wouldn't be sustainable long term. I found the food I ate tasty, healthy and easy to prepare. Though I had intended eating the same meals as Paul in the evenings, in fact he ended up eating from my menu often, instead, and enjoyed these meals! I do think my tastebuds have changed; I favour more fruit and salads now.

'As far as the exercise went, I carried on with the gym and the weekly run but walked for 40 minutes on the other days.

'I am sure this programme was the "missing link" that made it all happen. I need to see results to keep motivated.'

At the start, Pam's Body Mass Index was over the recommended maximum of 25 – losing nearly 12 lb has brought her BMI down to 24.5, well within health guidelines. She'd like to lose a few more pounds and firm up even more. And the good news is that she is back in work and looking forward to her life with renewed zest.

the healthy fast food plan

So you like 'fast food' and you don't want to give it up. Or your lifestyle is so unavoidably busy, that even if you want to, you can't.

But you're overweight and you need to lose those pounds. So how can you reconcile snacking, convenience foods, and little time to spend in the kitchen with slimming?

It **CAN** be done – with a bit of know-how. And here's where to find that knowledge.

In fact, many foods that are quick and easy to prepare (or need no preparation at all) are, actually, healthy and good for you, and not as high in fat and calories as you might think. So to start with, just to cheer you up and put you in a positive frame of mind, here are my top 20 quick and easy foods that you can eat without guilt on your slimming plan:

- Bread
- Most breakfast cereals
- Bananas
- Pasta
- Ready-made soup
- Potatoes
- Eggs
- Strawberries and cream
- Dried fruit
- Steak
- Cheese
- Baked beans
- Rice
- Baked potatoes
- Pizza
- Curry
- Chinese meals
- Ready-made sandwiches
- Burgers
- Chips

There are also plenty of other foods which you probably already consider 'healthy' or 'slimming' but which you don't see as fast food that will fit in with your lifestyle – fruits, salads, vegetables, yogurts, pulses and so on. In this plan, I aim to show you that these are all legitimate and tasty contributors towards a quick and easy diet.

And then, of course, there are the items that many people eat too much of when they live on snacks and fast food – chocolate, biscuits, cakes, crisps, ready desserts, take-aways and fried foods. I am going to show you how to incorporate these tastes and textures into your life while you slim.

Why snacking isn't a sin!

People who haven't much time to spend on their diet often say to me that they feel guilty for snacking rather than having just three 'proper' meals a day.

In fact, there is no need to worry about eating more than three times a day – it is the **RIGHT** way to eat! All research shows that eating 'little and often' is healthier than the 'let's just have one meal a day' syndrome. Our digestive systems cope better with smaller, frequent meals; our metabolic rate burns slightly quicker on such a regime, and when we're trying to slim and cut down calories, hunger pangs are much easier to keep at bay if a plan that allows snacks is followed.

The thing to alter is, of course, the type of snacks you are eating. A recent survey found that chocolate bars and crisps are this country's two most favoured snacks. On pages 59–67 you will find a whole range of ideas for tasty, quick snacks with which you can replace these, and other favourite high-calorie snack foods.

The Healthy Fast Food Plan allows you plenty of scope for both new snacks – and some of your old favourites!

Tips for healthy fast food shopping, cooking and eating

As any time management consultant will tell you, it is much quicker to be organised than to be disorganised, and that applies to your eating habits as much as anything else.

Many people who rely on fast food because they are so busy tend to grab what they can at the last minute; spend precious lunch breaks queuing for 'fast' food which turns out to be slower than making a packed lunch; spend valuable after-work time dashing out from home to the local supermarket or take-away because there's nothing in the refrigerator to eat – and so on.

Disorganised eating not only takes longer in the long run – it is also more likely to be the high-calorie eating that has helped you to put on a stone or more. You really need to plan ahead for your food, however busy you are. One hour one day a week spent planning ahead and shopping for what you need really **WILL** save you time and many, many calories each and every week. If you are reading this saying 'I can't', then please turn back to Chapter 1 and read what we discussed about the importance of your body in the scheme of things!

Getting Organised

Once a week

- Take 10 minutes to plan your diet. Check through Week 1 of this programme and decide which meal options you're going to go for. You will see that every lunchtime, you have a choice of a Packed Lunch, a Home Lunch, or a Takeout. In the evenings you have a choice of a Make-Ahead Meal (quick-to-make recipes that will chill or freeze until needed), a Real Meal in Moments, or a Ready Meal. Decide in conjunction with your diary if necessary. (For example, plan to have a Make-Ahead evening meal or Ready Meal on a night when you will be late home, rather than a meal you cook from scratch, albeit a quick one.) As you do so, start a shopping list for any meals or snacks that you can prepare or will be eating at home. Have different sections for fruit, vegetables, meat and fish, canned goods, chilled goods, drinks, frozen food, etc. Also stock up on handy store-cupboard items which are a boon to busy people – pastas, rice, canned pulses, tomato sauces and passata, preserves, oriental sauces and so on. Keep all the sections in the order in which your favourite or most convenient store is laid out, which will save time when you shop.

- Take 30 minutes to shop. If you're shopping just for you it won't take more than this. When shopping, remember time is money and if time is your precious commodity rather than cash, go for labour-saving products such as ready-peeled fruit, ready-washed and bagged mixed salad, ready-diced meats, ready-peeled vegetables and so on. All these items will make you more inclined to eat healthily. Choose fresh produce with the latest 'sell-by' date so it will keep for longer at home.
- Take 5 minutes to put everything away tidily where it will be easy to find when you want it. Store fruits, vegetables and salad in the refrigerator. Most items will keep well for up to a week if correctly stored. If foods for the freezer, such as chicken portions and bread, can be split up into one-portion sizes, do so before freezing; they will be much more convenient this way when it is time to defrost – and there is less chance of you eating more than you need.

When you have a little spare time

- Take a few minutes to prepare your Make-Ahead evening meal(s), if chosen. Cover and put in refrigerator. If you can make double the quantity and freeze the other half, this will save you even more time.

Before bed

- If you are having a packed lunch, take a few minutes to make that before you go to bed and pop it in the refrigerator too.

Cooking Tips

When preparing Make-Ahead Meals or Real Meals in Moments you can save a lot more time with these tips.

- If using the grill, put it on first to begin heating up while you do any necessary ingredient preparation.
- Always follow recipe instructions in the right order; they are designed to be time-saving.
- Get into the habit of using the microwave more for things like cooking chicken, fish, baked potatoes, quickly. It may be quicker to use hob and saucepan for vegetables.
- Many of the Meals in Moments and all the Make-Aheads can be frozen – so if you have time, make double the quantity and freeze the surplus.

Now read on for your instructions on following the Healthy Fast Food Plan, which includes a week to a page diet, snack ideas and recipes.

Every day of every week on the diet, YOU PICK:

- *A Breakfast* (some of which can be packed and eaten mid-morning if you prefer)
- *A Lunch* Choose either a Packed Lunch, a Home Lunch (some hot, some cold), or Takeout option (food from sandwich bars, etc.). Try to limit a Takeout option to once or twice a week.
- *An Evening Meal* Choose either a Make-Ahead Meal (easy things you can cook in spare minutes and freeze or keep chilled until required); a Real Meal in Moments (suppers that can be on the table in between 10 and 20 minutes of starting the preparation); or a Ready Meal (which is either a commercial chilled or frozen meal or a take-away). Try to limit Ready Meals to once or twice a week.

- *A Fruit Snack* Every day choose one portion of fruit of your choice. If choosing banana, make it a small one. Occasionally you can have a 125ml glass of fruit juice instead; try to make this a chilled fresh juice rather than the long-life variety – dilute it with sparkling mineral water for a longer drink.
- *Milk allowance* Have 250ml skimmed milk or 200ml semi-skimmed milk for use in tea and coffee or as a drink on its own. If not required, have 200ml low-fat natural bio yogurt instead – you need the calcium. Milk for breakfast cereals is on top of this allowance.
- *Snack Swaps* Every day choose 150 calories' worth of Snacks from the Snack Swaps on pages 50–1. Make these up as you like – e.g. six tiny 25-calorie snacks, one 100-calorie snack plus a 50, or whatever. If you have more than a stone to lose you can choose 200 calories' worth instead.

Unlimiteds

Every day you can have the following items in more or less unlimited quantity, though do try to go easy on artificially sweetened fizzy drinks and strong coffee.

- *Drinks* Tap water, mineral water, calorie-free drinks, weak tea or coffee (with milk from allowance, no sugar, use artificial sweeteners if necessary), herbal teas, green tea.
- *Food* Leafy green vegetables, green beans, runner beans, salad leaves, tomatoes, onion, courgettes, cucumber, celery, leeks, carrot, broccoli, cauliflower, aubergine, green peppers, yellow peppers – all raw or steamed, microwaved or boiled. Choose fresh or frozen and try to include as many of these as you can in your daily diet. They help fill you up and provide vitamins and minerals as well as fibre.

NOTE *Peas, broad beans, sweetcorn, red peppers and beetroot are higher in calories because they contain more sugar or starch and should be eaten in smaller quantities, if choosing instead of the 'Unlimited' vegetables.*

- *Condiments* Fresh or dried herbs and spices, lemon juice, Worcestershire sauce, light soy sauce, tomato purée, passata, vinegar, low-fat stock cubes and garlic.

Week's Treats

Every week on the plan you can also have your Week's Treats. Have **ONE** of the following to use as and when you like during the week (with the exception of the alcohol, which should not be consumed all in one evening – spread it over 2–3 evenings at least). Keep strictly to the amounts of these treats given as they are high-calorie foods.

- *wine* 1 whole bottle of dry white or red wine, maximum alcohol by volume 12 per cent.
- *beer or lager or cider* Five half pints standard strength or ten half pints low alcohol.
- *crisps* Three bags standard crisps or similar (maximum weight 30g each).
- *chocolate* Two bars 4-finger KitKat or standard Dairy Milk or Flyte **OR** Five Lo (not Gold) or Halo bars.
- *desserts* Five any ready desserts calorie-counted on the pack at 100 or less per dessert (e.g. some of Boots Shapers range, many individual chocolate mousses).

Men

Have $\frac{1}{3}$ larger portions of bread potatoes, pasta, etc. than those given and extra milk as liked.

SNACK SWAPS for Hungry Slimmers

Within the plan you are allowed up to 150 calories' worth of Snack Swaps every day (if you have a stone or less to lose) or 200 (if you have more than a stone to lose). The Snack Swaps can be mixed and matched as you will to add up to that daily total. It might be an idea to carry round an insulated bag or small box containing your Snack Swaps, or keep them in the kitchen or your office desk, so that you always have a snack to hand when you want something to eat – fast.

If you feel like something **SWEET** instead of chocolates, sweets or ice cream, choose . . .

For **25 calories** or less	For **50 calories** or less	For **100 calories** or less
• 3 ready-to-eat dried apricots • 1 ready tub sugar-free jelly • 1 Melba toast with low-sugar jam • 1 ripe plum	• 1 good handful Choco Krispies • 1 Jaffa cake • 1 sachet instant hot chocolate • 1 French Toast with runny honey • 1 dark rye Ryvita spread with 1 tsp Nutella • 1 peach, pear or orange	• 2-biscuit pack Weight Watchers Cookies • 1 Shape Twinpot yogurt • 1 Quaker Harvest Apple and Raisin Chewy Bar • 1 Boots Forest Fruit cereal bar • 1 ready tub low-fat rice pudding • 1 Häagen-Dazs frozen yogurt bar

If you feel like something **CRUNCHY** instead of high-fat crisps and other savoury snacks, choose . . .

For **25 calories** or less	For **50 calories** or less	For **100 calories** or less
• 1 dark rye Ryvita • 1 Slice a Rice • 2 fresh carrots • 2 pieces Melba toast	• 1 dark rye Ryvita with 1 tsp crunchy peanut butter • 1 Pogens Crisproll with Marmite • 1 Sharwood's Ready to Eat Poppadom crisps • 15g dry All-Bran (try it – it is delicious!) • 1 crisp apple • 2 sesame Grissini sticks	• 23g pack Butterkist popcorn • 1 pack Boots Shapers Potato Waffles • 1 pack Golden Lights Crisps • 1 pack Weight Watchers Weavers

If you want something **SAVOURY** or **CHEESY** instead of greasy chips or a high-fat chunk of Cheddar, try . . .

For **25 calories** or less	For **50 calories** or less	For **100 calories** or less
• Spring onions dipped in Waistline Salsa dressing • 2 tablespoons cold baked beans • I slice Melba toast with I tsp Philly Light or Marmite • I slice Melba toast with I sachet 10-calorie soup • I slice Melba toast spread with Kraft Free Choice mayo and chopped onion Triangle	• Carrot sticks dipped in Kraft Free Choice mayo • I Babybel Light individual cheese • I Cheestring • I Grissini stick with ⅓ pot Iceland Tuna Sweetcorn Dip • I dark rye Ryvita with I Kerrygold Light Cheese	• 100g cold cooked new potatoes sprinkled with sea salt • I mini pitta with 40g ready tzatziki • I × 20g pack Go Ahead Baked Potato Chips, cheese and onion I mini pitta dipped in 2 tbsp light fromage frais mixed with I level tbsp grated Parmesan cheese • I × 25g bag Twiglets

If you want something **SPICY**, forget the take-away curry or chilli . . .

For **25 calories** or less	For **50 calories** or less	For **100 calories** or less
• Spring onions dipped into Kraft Free Choice mayo laced with chilli powder	• I dark rye Ryvita spread with ¼ jar Boots Chilli Bean Spread • I Slice a Rice topped with plenty of ready hot and spicy salsa • I Sharwood's Ready to Eat large spiced poppadom with I tbsp ready salsa	• I mini pitta sliced with ⅓ of an 85g pot Iceland BBQ dip • 150g pot Uncle Ben's Hot Salsa with 4 slices Melba toast • I pack Boots Shapers Indonesian style crackers

If you want something **STARCHY**, leave the gateau or the doughnut and go for . . .

For **25 calories** or less	For **50 calories** or less	For **100 calories** or less
• I Amaretti biscuit • I tsp cooked rice	• I Jaffa cake • Slice of Sunblest Danish White with a little low-fat spread	• I mini white pitta with I tsp low-sugar jam • Average slice bread from large sliced loaf with low-fat spread and low-sugar jam • Round crumpet with low-fat spread • Medium slice malt loaf with low-fat spread • I large banana

WEEK ONE

Notes

- For instructions, allowances and 'unlimiteds', see pages 48–9.
- Don't forget to add unlimited vegetable and salad items to your meals whenever you can.
- Don't forget to fill up on your daily Snack Swaps and your daily Fruit Snack.
- Don't forget your Week's Treats too!
- When **BREAD** is mentioned in the diet, unless otherwise stated it is a slice from a medium-cut large sliced loaf.
- If **FRUIT** is mentioned within a meal but not specified, choose any fresh, frozen or canned in juice fruit which can be either 1 whole medium fruit, 2 small fruits, 1 small banana, a large bowlful of berries, a small bowlful of mixed fruit salad or a ringpull can of Fruitini. Do not use dried fruit unless specified and avoid fruit canned in syrup.
- You will be pleased to see that weighing and measuring have been avoided when possible through the use of single-portion items, and spoons.

Choose one meal from each section every day.

Breakfasts

- Shape diet fruit yogurt; 1 apple; 1 slice bread with a little low-fat spread and low-sugar jam, marmalade or Marmite.
- Medium bowl (25g) branflakes or cornflakes, Special K, Just Right or All-Bran with skimmed milk to cover; fruit.
- 125g pot natural low-fat bio yogurt with small handful no added sugar or salt muesli and fruit.
- ½ can wholewheat spaghetti in tomato sauce on 1 slice toasted bread, with a little low-fat spread.
- 1 Shape Bio Twinpot yogurt, any variety; 1 large banana.

Lunches Packed

- 2 slices bread with a little low-fat spread filled with 1 individual portion Bel Paese cream cheese or 2 slices extra-lean ham, 2 teaspoons sweet pickle, lettuce; 1 Shape fruit fromage frais; 1 portion fruit.
- 1 white pitta filled with 1 × 100g can tuna in brine, drained, mixed with 1 tablespoon Kraft Free Choice mayonnaise and chopped crisp raw vegetables/salad of choice; 1 Shape fruit yogurt.

Lunches Home

- ½ 400g can baked beans in tomato sauce on 1 slice toast, with a little low-fat spread, topped with 1 level tablespoon grated half-fat cheese; 1 large banana.
- 1 Findus French Bread Pizza, ham and pineapple or cheese and tomato flavour; Shape fruit fromage frais; fruit.
- Ten-calorie soup (optional); cooked chicken breast portion with unlimited salad items of choice; small wholemeal roll and low-fat spread.

Lunches Takeout

- Any supermarket calorie-counted sandwich 300 calories or less; fruit.
- McDonald's hamburger (regular, no cheese); McDonald's pure orange juice.

Evening Meals Make-Ahead Meals

- Tarragon Pork (see recipe page 63).
- Chicken and Mushroom Pancakes (see recipe page 62).

Evening Meals Real Meals in Moments

- If you have any leftover cooked potatoes plus eggs – Spanish Omelette (see recipe page 66)
- 1 average turkey fillet, grilled or fried using a little Fry Light spray in a non-stick pan; large portion frozen mixed vegetables; 4 tablespoons mashed potato (instant if liked, or mashed using skimmed milk); 1 dessertspoon relish of choice.
- 50g (dry weight) couscous, reconstituted according to pack instructions and topped with 1 whole 340–400g can ratatouille plus 2 tablespoons grated Parmesan cheese.

Evening Meals Ready Meals

(Do have plenty of your unlimited vegetable/salad with any selection from here.)
- Findus Dinner Supreme Chicken Curry.
- St Michael Cannelloni (285g).
- Birds Eye Roast Beef Platter.
- Birds Eye MenuMaster Macaroni Cheese.

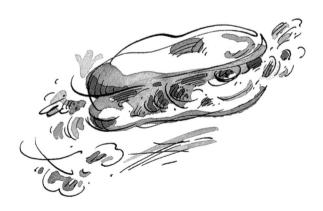

WEEK TWO

Notes

As Week 1 plus:
- Don't forget to read through your meal options and plan ahead for the week. It'll save you time and hunger!

Breakfasts

- 1 pot of Müller Crunch Corner bio yogurt Honey and Muesli.
- 2 slices bread or toast with low-fat spread and low-sugar jam or marmalade or Marmite.
- 2 Weetabix with skimmed milk to cover; 1 small glass grapefruit juice.
- 125ml low-fat natural bio yogurt; 1 small banana; 1 teaspoon honey.

Lunches Packed

- 2 slices bread spread with Kraft Free Choice mayonnaise and filled with unlimited salad plus 2 slices lean turkey from vacuum pack, 2 tsp cranberry sauce (optional); 1 Prewett's Banana bar.
- 3 dark rye Ryvitas with a little low-fat spread; 1 Camembert triangle (pick and mix size); 1 tomato; 1 apple; 200g pot Müller Light yogurt.

Lunches Home

- 1 whole carton New Covent Garden Tomato or Lentil and Tomato soup; 1 slice bread with low-fat spread.
- Large egg poached on 1 slice toast with low-fat spread; 2 satsumas; Quaker Harvest Chewy bar.

Lunches Takeout

- Take-away baked potato with baked bean filling; fruit.
- Small baguette or soft wholemeal bap filled with chicken and salad (no mayonnaise).
- Tesco Roast Vegetable Baguette; kiwi or satsuma or plum.

Evening Meals Make-Ahead Meals

- Balti Curry (see recipe page 64)
- Penne Primavera (see recipe page 66)

Evening Meals Real Meals in Moments

- Individual portion frozen cod fillet in breadcrumbs, grilled; 100g pack McCain Micro Chips, heated in microwave; grilled tomato; 3 tablespoons frozen petit pois or peas, boiled or microwaved.
- If you have a selection of sweet peppers – Stir-fried Peppers and Egg (see recipe page 67).
- Pitta pizza – Heat grill; spread 1 tablespoon sundried tomato paste or some ready-made Italian Tomato Sauce over one side of a pitta bread; top with sliced tomato and finely chopped onion and seasoning, and top that with 2 level tablespoons grated half-fat mozzarella (available in resealable freezable packs). Grill until bubbling and serve with salad.

Evening Meals Ready Meals

- Indian take-away vegetable curry with plain boiled rice.
- Chilled or frozen individual size Fisherman's Pie (about 300g), salad, 2 tablespoons peas.
- Weight Watchers Beef Lasagne; salad.

WEEK THREE

Notes

As Week I plus:

- If you like you can choose a meal option from another week – as long as you swap breakfast for breakfast, lunch for lunch, and so on.
- Don't forget to take plenty of exercise.

Breakfasts

- Large boiled egg; I slice bread or toast with a little low-fat spread; small glass grapefruit juice.
- I individual box Kelloggs' cereal from pick and mix selection with skimmed milk to cover; fruit.
- I Nutri-Grain morning bar; I Shape fruit yogurt or I portion fruit.

Lunches Packed

- 2 slices bread with a little low-fat spread filled with 2 slices lean chicken from vacuum pack and salad plus I dessertspoon Kraft Free Choice mayonnaise; I large banana.
- I can of John West Tuna Light Meal; I Shape fromage frais; I portion fruit.

Lunches At home

- 275g baked potato filled with 100g pot ready-made tzatziki; salad or fruit.
- ½ medium ripe avocado filled with oil-free French dressing or a dash of balsamic vinegar; salad; I small wholemeal roll with a little low-fat spread; I Shape fruit yogurt.

Lunches Takeout

- I portion pasta salad with mushrooms and tomato sauce.
- I reduced-calorie sandwich 300 calories or less; I portion fruit.

Evening Meals Make-Ahead Meals

- Salmon with Pesto and Spaghetti (see recipe page 59).
- Sweet and Sour Pork and Noodles (see recipe page 64).

Evening Meals Real Meals in Moments

- From the store-cupboard – Pasta with Sardines and Sultanas (see recipe page 59).
- Chicken tacos – slice I chicken breast fillet and microwave or stir-fry in Old El Paso mild or hot taco sauce until cooked through; use to fill 2 taco shells with chopped crisp lettuce, tomato, onion. Top with I tablespoon ready-made guacamole (avocado purée/dip)* or with I tablespoon Greek yogurt or half-fat crème fraîche.

Evening Meals Ready Meals

- Sharwood's frozen Balti Vegetable curry with Naan bread; I dessertspoon sweet mango chutney; fruit.
- St Michael Jacket Potato with Fresh Cauliflower and Broccoli; I tablespoon grated half-fat Cheddar over top; fruit or Shape fruit yogurt.
- Ross frozen Tikka Chicken (340g); I dessertspoon mango chutney; salad.
- ½ average 2-portion cheese and tomato pizza.

* FROM DELI COUNTER OR IN JARS FROM MOST SUPERMARKETS.

WEEK **FOUR**

Notes

As Week I plus:

- If you have to eat in a restaurant during the Plan, check out the tips in the Business Plan (see page 128), and if you feel you've eaten too much, go for a day or two without your Snack Swaps.

Breakfasts

- Individual sachet or box muesli with milk from allowance; fruit.
- Pot of French-style fruit yogurt; large banana.
- Fruit Compôte (see recipe page 43) with 125ml pot low-fat natural bio yogurt.

Lunches Packed

- Pitta bread filled with I can John West Tuna in Italian tomato sauce plus extra chopped salad.
- Sandwich of 2 slices bread with a little low-fat spread filled with 40g half-fat Cheddar, tomato, cucumber; Boots Shapers yogurt mousse.

Lunches Home

- Unlimited fresh tomatoes, halved and grilled or stir-fried in Fry Light spray in a non-stick pan, seasoned, on 2 slices toast with a little low-fat spread and topped with I tablespoon half-fat Cheddar or mozzarella; I large banana.
- Full can of Heinz Chicken with Pasta and Vegetables soup; wholemeal bap with a little low-fat spread; fruit.

Lunches Takeout

- St Michael Lite Layered Egg Salad; fruit; Shape fromage frais.
- Boots Shapers triple sandwich pack, any variety; fruit.
- Tesco Chinese Style Chicken Salad Bowl; fruit.

Evening Meals Make-Ahead Meals

- Chicken Curry (see recipe page 62).
- Shepherd's Pie (see recipe page 65).

Evening Meals Real Meals in Moments

- If you have some fresh mushrooms – boil 50g (dry weight) pasta shapes of choice and while they are cooking, slice and stir-fry 100g firm tasty mushrooms (e.g. chestnuts) or oyster mushrooms in I dessertspoon corn oil, then add $\frac{1}{3}$ jar of Italian tomato sauce with chilli or herbs, stir to heat through and serve over the pasta with I level tablespoon Parmesan on top; salad; fruit.
- Tuna and Vegetable Stir-fry (see recipe page 60).
- Medium salmon steak, grilled or dry-fried; 150g canned or frozen new potatoes; good portion frozen peas or petit pois; I dessertspoon ready-made hollandaise sauce *or* light mayonnaise.

Evening Meals Ready Meals

- Birds Eye Vegetarian Indian Meal.
- Findus Potato and Ham Gratin.
- Prawn Chop Suey from Chinese take-away.

WEEK **FIVE**

Notes

As Week 1

Breakfasts

- Nutri-Grain bar; fruit.
- English muffin with a little low-fat spread and low-sugar jam or marmalade.
- Medium bowlful instant porridge made with skimmed milk and water; 1 teaspoon syrup or brown sugar or honey; fruit.

Lunches Packed

- Tuna Pâté (see recipe page 60) inside 2 slices bread with a little low-fat spread plus salad; fruit.
- 175g leftover cooked rice mixed with 1 handful (50g) cold chopped chicken or ham plus chopped crisp raw vegetables, etc., chopped dried apricots and oil-free French dressing; Shape fruit yogurt.

Lunches Home

- 1 × St Michael 95 per cent Fat-Free Stonebake Vegetable Pizza; salad.
- Small (75g) baguette with a little low-fat spread; 40g half-fat Cheddar; 2 teaspoons pickle; salad.
- 205g can Heinz Curried Beans with Sultanas on 1 slice toast with a little low-fat spread.

Lunches Takeout

- Boots Shapers Lunchtime Selection; fruit.
- St Michael Pasta and Chargrilled Chicken Salad; 1 banana.
- McDonald's McChicken Sandwich.

Evening Meals Make-Ahead Meals

- Aubergine and Lentil Curry (see recipe page 111).
- Nasi Goreng (see recipe page 67).

Evening Meals Real Meals in Moments

- Swordfish and Red Pepper Kebabs (see recipe page 60).
- Turkey with Egg Thread Noodles (see recipe page 63).
- Corned beef hash – blend together 100g corned beef and 150g ready-made potato (e.g. instant) and fry in a little Fry Light in a non-stick pan until golden on both sides; serve with 4 tablespoons baked beans.

Evening Meals Ready Meals

- Sainsbury's Creamy Leek and Mushroom Bake; salad.
- St Michael Tagliatelle with Chicken, Tomato and Basil.
- Birds Eye Chicken Chasseur.
- St Michael Tuna and Pasta Bake.

WEEK SIX

Notes

As Week I plus:

- When you've finished the plan and reached your target weight, turn to Chapter 10 for more information on keeping the weight off for good.

Breakfasts

- 6 tablespoons baked beans on I slice toast with a little low-fat spread.
- Müller Fruit Corner yogurt; small glass grapefruit juice.
- Individual box cornflakes from pick and mix; skimmed milk to cover; small fruit.

Lunches Packed

- Hard-boiled medium egg; 3 dark rye Ryvitas with a little low-fat spread; medium banana; French-style fruit yogurt.
- I × 43g can dressed crab in 2 slices bread with low-fat spread plus lettuce and cucumber; fruit; I Shape fromage frais.

Lunches Home

- Small can butter beans, drained and mixed with sliced tomato, onion and $\frac{1}{2}$ avocado or I × 100g can tuna in brine or water, drained; I slice bread with low-fat spread; fruit.
- Can Weight Watchers soup, any variety; wholemeal roll and a little low-fat spread; Camembert triangle from pick and mix; plum.

Lunches Takeout

- Any ready sandwich 300 calories or less; fruit or I Shape fromage frais.
- Boots Balti Prawn or Mexican Flatbread; Boots Shapers Melon Cocktail; 125g tub low-fat natural bio yogurt.

Evening Meals Make-Ahead Meals

- Salmon and Vegetable Medley (see recipe page 61).
- Moroccan Lamb with Couscous (see recipe page 65).

Evening Meals Real Meals in Moments

- Chicken Tikka Kebabs (see recipe page 62).
- Sautéed Mussels (see recipe page 61).
- If you have some frozen prawns, spring onions and a 100g jar of sweet and sour sauce – defrost 125g prawns in warm water for a few minutes, drain. In a saucepan, heat the sauce with the prawns and chopped spring onions. Serve on 50g (dry weight) couscous which you have reconstituted while the prawns are cooking.
- 2-egg omelette cooked in non-stick pan with a little Fry Light and filled with 30g lean ham; I × 100g pack McCain Micro Chips; salad.

Evening Meals Ready Meals

- St Michael Chicken and Pasta Bake.
- Findus Dinner Supreme Toad in the Hole.
- Birds Eye Healthy Options Vegetable Indian Meal.

20 QUICK AND EASY RECIPES

PASTA WITH SARDINES AND SULTANAS

(Real Meals in Moments, Week 3)
10 minutes to prepare and cook.

Serves 1
470 calories and 21g fat per portion

40g (dry weight) spaghettini or other thin pasta

1 dessertspoon olive oil

2 spring onions, sliced into thin rounds

4 canned sardines, well drained and dried with
    kitchen paper

1 level tablespoon sultanas

1 level dessertspoon pine nuts

A dash of lemon juice

1 tablespoon fresh parsley or 1 teaspoon freeze-dried

A little salt and black pepper

Boil some water in a kettle and fill a saucepan, bring back to boil; add the pasta and a dash of salt. Boil, uncovered, for 10 minutes or as pack instructs.

Meanwhile, heat the oil in a small non-stick frying pan and stir in the onions. Chop the sardines each into four and when the onions are slightly soft, add them to the pan with the sultanas and pine nuts. Stir very gently for a minute, adding the lemon juice, parsley and seasoning half way through. When the pasta is ready, drain and serve with the sardine sauce lightly combined.

SALMON WITH PESTO AND SPAGHETTI

(Make-Ahead Meal, Week 3)
25 minutes to prepare and cook; will freeze

Serves 2
402 calories and 16.5g fat per portion

175g salmon fillet

Fry Light spray

1 large red pepper

1 × 250g pack Napolina Creamy Tomato and Pesto
    Sauce

80g (dry weight) tagliatelle or spaghetti

Basil leaves, to garnish (optional)

Heat a medium non-stick frying pan (which has a lid) sprayed well with Fry Light. Chop the salmon into bite-sized cubes and add to the pan, stirring gently until lightly golden. Remove with a slotted spoon and set aside. Deseed and thinly slice the pepper and stir for 2 minutes in the pan with more Fry Light added. Add the sauce to the pan, turn the heat down and simmer, covered, for 20 minutes or until the peppers are fairly tender. Add the salmon for the last 2 minutes of cooking.

Meanwhile, cook the tagliatelle in boiling salted water and drain.

Arrange the pasta in two freezerproof, microwaveproof lidded single-serving dishes and top with the sauce. To serve, reheat in the microwave until piping hot and garnish with fresh basil if liked.

TUNA PÂTÉ

(Packed Lunches, Week 5)
2 minutes to prepare; will freeze

Serves 2
153 calories and 5.3g fat per portion

125g can smoked tuna in oil, drained
50g fat-free fromage frais
50g Kraft Free Choice mayonnaise
1 small onion, very finely chopped
1 dessertspoon tomato purée
1 teaspoon lemon juice
Black pepper

In a large bowl, beat together all the ingredients until you have a rough pâté. Chill, covered, until needed. (Can be chilled or frozen in individual ramekins if you like.)

Use for sandwich filling (see Week 5); starter; lunch with crispbreads and salad.

TUNA AND VEGETABLE STIR-FRY

(Real Meals in Moments, Week 4)
15 minutes to prepare and cook; will freeze

Serves 1
435 calories and 12.5g fat per portion

100g mixed peppers (see note)
1 dessertspoon corn or olive oil
40g quick-cook rice
1 medium leek or 3 spring onions
125g fresh tuna
One-third of a 160g jar of St Michael Tomato, Basil and
    Oregano cook-in sauce

Deseed and chop the peppers while the oil is heating in a non-stick pan. Add them and stir-fry for 7–8 minutes.

Meanwhile cook the rice according to pack instructions.

Thinly slice the leek or onions into rounds, and when the peppers are fairly soft, add them to the pan and stir for 2 minutes. Slice the tuna into thin strips and add to the pan, stirring for 2 more minutes. Add the sauce to the pan and heat through. Serve with the rice.

NOTE *To save time preparing the peppers yourself (and because to get a good mix of colours you would need to buy a lot more than you need for this recipe), ready-sliced mixed peppers in resealable bags can sometimes be bought from the freezer section of the supermarket. Otherwise you could use peppers canned in brine, well drained, which would then not need stir-frying for more than a minute.*

SWORDFISH AND RED PEPPER KEBABS

(Real Meals in Moments, Week 5)
15 minutes to prepare and cook

Serves 1
425 calories and 19g fat per portion

25g (dry weight) couscous
150g swordfish fillet
1 small red pepper
1 teaspoon olive oil
100g chopped canned tomatoes
½ teaspoon garlic purée
Salt and black pepper
15g blanched ground almonds

Reconstitute the couscous according to pack instructions (usually, pour boiling water over and leave to stand for 10 minutes).

Meanwhile, heat the grill and chop the swordfish into bite-sized cubes; deseed and chop the pepper into squares, and thread the swordfish and pepper pieces onto a kebab. Brush with the oil. Grill for 8 minutes, turning once.

While the kebab is cooking, whizz the tomatoes, garlic purée and seasoning in a blender and stir in the almonds to make a rich sauce. Serve the kebab on the couscous with the sauce.

SALMON AND VEGETABLE MEDLEY

(Make-Ahead Meals, Week 6)
20 minutes to prepare and cook; will freeze

Serves 2
396 calories and 18g fat per portion

160g new potatoes, ready cleaned
2 small to medium carrots (about 100g)
100g broccoli
Fry Light spray
50g frozen peas
2 small leeks (about 100g), cut into very thin rounds
160g salmon fillet, cut into small pieces
Half a pack Napolina Creamy Pasta Bake for Lasagne (see note)
2 level tablespoons packet croûtons, crushed
1 level tablespoon grated Parmesan cheese

Cut the potatoes into bite-sized chunks if necessary and boil for 15 minutes or until all the pieces are tender; drain.

Meanwhile, cut the carrots and broccoli into thin slices, heat a non-stick frying pan coated with Fry Light and stir-fry the carrots and broccoli vigorously for 2 minutes. Add the rest of the ingredients except the breadcrumbs and cheese, stir well and simmer for 15 minutes. Stir the drained potatoes into the pan.

Spoon the mixture into two lidded individual freezerproof, ovenproof and microwaveproof containers and sprinkle the crumbs and cheese on top before chilling or freezing. Reheat in the microwave or oven until piping hot and flash under grill if liked.

NOTE *The remainder of the lasagne sauce will freeze.*

SAUTÉED MUSSELS

(Real Meals in Moments, Week 6)
15 minutes to prepare and cook

Serves 1
417 calories and 12.5g fat per portion

450g ready-prepared mussels in their shells
10g (1 level dessertspoon) butter
1 small onion
50ml dry white wine
Fresh parsley (optional)
1 teaspoon fresh chilled garlic purée or 1 crushed clove garlic
Juice of ½ lemon
100g canned chopped tomatoes with herbs
Salt and black pepper
60g piece French bread

Check over the mussels and discard any that are broken or cracked. Heat the butter in a large non-stick frying pan; finely chop the onion and stir-fry it over a medium high heat until softened. Pour in the wine and bubble for a minute, then add the parsley, if using, garlic, lemon juice, chopped tomatoes and seasoning; stir well and bring to a simmer. Add the mussels, cover the pan and cook for a few minutes, stirring once or twice, or until all the mussel shells have opened. If any haven't opened, discard them before serving with the French bread to dip in the juices.

CHICKEN AND MUSHROOM PANCAKES

(Make-Ahead Meals, Week 1)
10 minutes to prepare and cook; will freeze

Serves 2
445 calories and 14g fat per portion

200g stir-fry lean chicken pieces
Fry Light spray
200g small firm tasty mushrooms
1 × 50g pack Knorr Parsley Sauce mix
100g frozen sweetcorn or petit pois, defrosted
    (see note)
Salt and pepper
4 medium ready-to-eat pancakes (see note)
Fresh parsley (optional)

Heat a non-stick frying pan sprayed with Fry Light and add the chicken in one layer. Leave until the underneath is golden, then turn the pieces over and repeat (if you try to stir them about until they are sealed, they will stick!).

Remove the pan from the heat. Cut the mushrooms into thin slices and make up the parsley sauce according to pack instructions. Add the sauce, mushrooms, sweetcorn and seasoning to the pan, stir well and bring to a simmer for 2–3 minutes. Spoon a quarter of the sauce into the middle of each pancake and roll up or fold into quarters.

Carefully place into one or two freezerproof, ovenproof/microwaveproof dish/es of suitable size, sprinkle with parsley if using and chill or freeze. Reheat in the microwave or oven until filling is bubbling.

NOTE *Sweetcorn or peas can be defrosted in moments either by placing in a sieve and running water over them, or in the microwave. Ready-made thin pancakes (crêpes) can be bought in packs from most supermarkets; find them near the breads. Any surplus pancakes can be frozen.*

CHICKEN TIKKA KEBABS

(Real Meals in Moments, Week 6)
kebabs and pitta will freeze but not the relish

Serves 1
395 calories and 8g fat per portion

120g lean chicken fillet
1 tablespoon 8 per cent fat fromage frais
1 good teaspoon mild curry paste
1 good teaspoon mango chutney
2cm piece cucumber, chopped
2 tablespoons natural whole-milk bio yogurt
½ teaspoon garlic purée
1 whole pitta bread

Heat the grill. Cut the chicken into bite-sized cubes. Mix together the fromage frais, curry paste and mango chutney in a bowl and add the chicken pieces to coat well. Thread the chicken onto a kebab and grill under a medium hot heat for 8 minutes or so until cooked through, turning once or twice.

Ffinely chop the cucumber and mix with the yogurt and garlic. Add the pitta to the grill for the last minute of cooking to heat through, turning once. Serve the kebab with the warm pitta and the yogurt relish.

CHICKEN CURRY

(Make-Ahead Meals, Week 4)
25 minutes to prepare and cook; will freeze

Serves 2
415 calories and 8g fat per portion

200g potatoes
100g broccoli florets or courgette slices
50g (dry weight) basmati rice

1 dessertspoon corn oil

1 medium onion

200g lean chicken boneless thighs

200g jar Sharwood's Basil and Chilli Stir-Fry Sauce

3 tablespoons low-fat natural bio yogurt

Peel the potatoes, cut them into bite-sized chunks and boil until tender, adding the broccoli or courgette for the last 3 minutes of cooking. Drain.

Meanwhile, cook the basmati rice in a little water according to pack instructions; reserve.

Heat the oil in a non-stick frying pan and while it is heating, slice the onion thinly and halve the slices. Add the onion to the pan and stir over a medium high heat until transparent and just turning golden. Cut the chicken into bite-sized slices and add to the pan, stirring again for a few minutes. Add the sauce and stir over medium heat for a few more minutes, adding a very little water if the mix seems too thick, then stir in the potatoes and broccoli and finally the rice. Spoon into two individual lidded freezerproof, ovenproof/microwaveproof containers and freeze or chill. Reheat until piping hot and serve with the yogurt drizzled over.

TURKEY WITH EGG THREAD NOODLES

(Real Meals in Moments, Week 5)
15 minutes to prepare and cook; will freeze

Serves 1
415 calories and 10.5g fat per portion

1 small green pepper

1 dessertspoon corn oil

40g (dry weight) medium egg thread noodles

100g turkey fillet

½ teaspoon garlic purée

¼ jar of Sharwood's Yellow Bean Sauce

1 dessertspoon light soy sauce

1 pinch ground chilli or dash chilli sauce

2 tablespoons chicken stock from cube mixed with
    1 level teaspoon cornflour

Deseed and thinly slice the pepper. Heat the oil in a non-stick frying pan and fry the pepper over a medium high heat, stirring from time to time, for 6–7 minutes.

Meanwhile, pour boiling water over the noodles and allow to stand for a few minutes until soft, drain and reserve.

Slice the turkey fillet and add to the frying pan, stirring for 3–4 minutes. Add the garlic purée, bean sauce, soy sauce and chilli and stir for a minute before adding the stock mixture. Stir again for 1 minute. Serve the pan mixture on the noodles. (If the noodles have cooled, you can add them to the frying pan and stir through with the sauce to reheat.)

If freezing, freeze in an individual lidded freezerproof, ovenproof/microwaveproof dish and reheat until piping hot all the way through.

TARRAGON PORK

(Make-Ahead Meals, Week 1)
15 minutes to prepare and cook; will freeze

Serves 2
382 calories and 14g fat per portion

75g pasta shapes of choice

1 dessertspoon corn oil

8 shallots, halved

225g pork tenderloin

25ml dry white wine

25ml full-fat crème fraîche

1 tablespoon fresh chopped tarragon
    (or 1 dessertspoon freeze-dried)

Salt and pepper

Boil a kettle of water and fill a saucepan, add the pasta with a little salt and cook until tender – about 12 minutes. Drain.

Meanwhile, heat the oil in a non-stick frying pan and add the shallots to fry, stirring from time to time, over a medium heat. Slice the pork tenderloin into 1cm thick slices and when the shallots are beginning to brown after about 5 minutes, add the pork to the pan. Cook to brown each side, then add the wine, lower the heat and simmer for 2–3 minutes. Add the crème fraîche, tarragon and seasoning, stir well and serve with the pasta.

BALTI CURRY

(Make-Ahead Meals, Week 2)
25 minutes to prepare and cook; will freeze

Serves 2
418 calories and 15g fat per portion

60g (dry weight) basmati rice

175g extra-lean minced beef

1 medium onion

1 small (about 150g) aubergine

2 whole tomatoes (canned, drained or fresh, skinned)

100g baby spinach or spring greens or French beans

200g Madhur Jaffrey or Sharwood's Balti Sauce

2 tablespoons low-fat natural yogurt

Put the rice on to simmer in a little lightly salted water according to pack instructions.

Meanwhile, put the meat in a non-stick frying pan and slowly heat, stirring from time to time, gradually increasing heat so that the fat runs out (which it will even with lean meat) and the meat begins to brown.

Meanwhile, finely slice and chop the onion. When the meat is browned, remove it from the pan with a slotted spoon and reserve. In the remaining fat, sauté the onion, stirring from time to time, until transparent and turning golden. While the onion is cooking, chop the aubergine into 1cm rounds and then each into a quarter, and quarter the tomatoes. Add both to the pan and stir-fry with the onions for a few minutes. Add the spinach to the pan and stir. (If using spring greens, shred them finely.) Return the meat to the pan with the sauce, stir, bring to a simmer and cook, stirring frequently, for a few minutes.

Spoon the cooked rice into two individual, freezerproof, ovenproof/microwaveproof lidded containers and spoon the curry on top. Freeze or chill and reheat thoroughly, before serving drizzled with the yogurt.

NOTE *Fresh coriander leaves sprinkled on top are very good. You can serve the Balti curry with mini pitta breads instead of the rice if you like, in which case you can add a dessertspoon of mango chutney per serving, if you want.*

SWEET AND SOUR PORK AND NOODLES

(Make-Ahead Meals, Week 3)
20 minutes to prepare and cook; will freeze

Serves 2
413 calories and 9g fat per portion

75g (dry weight) fine egg thread noodles

1 dessertspoon groundnut oil

1 medium onion or 6 spring onions, halved lengthways

200g lean pork fillet

1 medium carrot

1 small yellow pepper

50g Chinese leaves or Cos lettuce

50g beansprouts

160g jar Sharwood's Sweet and Sour Sauce

Pour boiling water over the noodles in a pan and leave to soften according to pack instructions; drain.

Meanwhile, heat the oil in non-stick frying pan and stir-fry the onion until turning golden. Cut the pork into thin strips and add it to the pan, stirring until brown. Slice the carrot and yellow pepper into thin strips and add to the pan, stirring again for a few minutes, adding a little water or chicken stock if the pan gets too dry. Add the Chinese leaves, beansprouts and sauce and stir for 2 minutes. Arrange the noodles in two individual, lidded, freezerproof, ovenproof/microwaveproof dishes and spoon the pork sauce on top. Freeze or chill. Reheat thoroughly.

NOTE *If you don't want to use beansprouts, increase the amount of Chinese leaves or Cos instead.*

SHEPHERD'S PIE

(Make-Ahead Meals, Week 4)
20 minutes to prepare and cook; will freeze

Serves 2
400 calories and 14g fat per portion

150g lean lamb mince
1 medium onion
100g baked beans in tomato sauce
50ml onion gravy
1 tablespoon tomato purée
1 teaspoon mixed herbs
400g (made-up weight) instant mashed potato
1 tablespoon grated Parmesan cheese

Put the mince evenly in a non-stick frying pan and slowly heat up, gradually increasing the heat so the fat runs out as the meat browns. Stir from time to time.

Meanwhile, finely chop the onion. When the meat is browned, remove with a slotted spoon, leaving the fat behind, and reserve. Now add the onion to the pan and stir-fry for a few minutes until soft. Return the meat to the pan with the baked beans, onion gravy, tomato purée and herbs, and stir well. Cook over a low heat for a few minutes and then spoon into a suitable dish or dishes. Smooth the mashed potato over the top evenly, sprinkle over the cheese and freeze or chill. To serve, defrost thoroughly and heat through in a conventional oven to brown the top, or microwave until hot and then flash under the grill.

MOROCCAN LAMB WITH COUSCOUS

(Make-Ahead Meals, Week 6)
25 minutes to prepare and cook excluding marinating time; will freeze

Serves 2
385 calories and 14.5g fat per portion

225g lean lamb fillet
25ml Lea and Perrin's Sundried Tomato and Herb Marinade
60g (dry weight) Sammy's Couscous with Sundried Tomatoes and Herbs
2 sweet peppers – red, orange or yellow or mix
1 teaspoon olive oil
Salt and pepper
3cm piece cucumber
3 tablespoons Greek yogurt

Up to 8 hours before you want to cook, cut the lamb into bite-sized pieces, place in a non-metallic bowl and pour the marinade over, coating well. Cover and leave in the refrigerator until cooking time.

At cooking time, reconstitute the couscous in boiling water for 6 minutes (you can use plain couscous if you like).

Meanwhile, heat the grill and quarter and deseed the peppers. Lay them on a baking tray and brush with the olive oil and season. Thread the lamb onto 2 kebabs. When the grill is hot, place both lamb and peppers under the grill. Grill the peppers until beginning to char and soften. Grill the kebabs for about 8 minutes, turning once and basting with any remaining marinade.

Meanwhile, chop the cucumber finely and mix with the yogurt. The peppers and the kebabs will be cooked at about the same time. Serve with the couscous and the yogurt relish.

PENNE PRIMAVERA

(Make-Ahead Meals, Week 2)
20 minutes to prepare and cook; will freeze

Serves 2
400 calories and 10g fat per portion

150g (dry weight) penne pasta tricolour
1 medium courgette
50g sugarsnap peas or baby sweetcorn
1 dessertspoon olive oil
2 medium leeks
100g firm mushrooms
1 teaspoon garlic purée
75ml passata
Salt and black pepper
2 level tablespoons half-fat crème fraîche
2 tablespoons grated Parmesan cheese

Cook the pasta in boiling, lightly salted water until cooked; drain.

Meanwhile, thinly slice the courgette and parboil the courgette slices and sugarsnaps or sweetcorn for 2 minutes, drain; pat dry on kitchen paper. Heat the oil in a non-stick frying pan. While it is heating, slice the leeks thinly, then add to the pan and stir until

beginning to soften. Thinly slice the mushrooms. Add the courgette, peas, mushrooms and garlic purée and stir for 2–3 minutes. Add the passata and seasoning and simmer for a further 2–3 minutes. Stir in the crème fraîche and then, when the pasta is cooked, mix the sauce with the pasta and top with the cheese. Spoon into two lidded individual, freezerproof ovenproof/microwaveproof containers and freeze or chill. Reheat thoroughly before serving.

SPANISH OMELETTE

(Real Meals in Moments, Week 1)
10 minutes to prepare and cook

Serves 1
408 calories and 18g fat per portion

2 large eggs
Salt and pepper
1 teaspoon corn or olive oil
100g leftover cooked potato
3 spring onions
1 slice bread, toasted with a little low-fat spread

In a bowl, beat the eggs with a little cold water and salt and pepper. Heat the oil in a small non-stick frying pan.

Meanwhile, slice the potato thinly and chop the spring onions. When the pan is hot, add the eggs to the pan and arrange the potato slices and onions around the pan evenly. Cook over a low to medium heat until the underside of the egg is golden. Flash the pan under the grill to brown the top or place an inverted plate over the top of the pan and turn the omelette over to cook the other side. Serve when both sides are set and golden, with the toast and plenty of salad.

STIR-FRIED PEPPERS AND EGG

(Real Meals in Moments, Week 2)
15 minutes to prepare and cook

Serves 1
395 calories and 19g fat per portion

1 tablespoon olive oil
200g mixed peppers
1 small onion
1 fresh tomato
1 pinch ground chilli
Salt and black pepper
1 large egg
1 mini pitta

Heat the olive oil in a medium non-stick frying pan.

Meanwhile, deseed the peppers and very thinly slice both them and the onion. Add to the pan and stir-fry for 7–8 minutes until soft and tinged golden. Chop the tomato (deseeded if you like) and add it to the pan with the chilli and seasoning. Poach the egg and heat the pitta. Serve the cooked pepper mixture topped with the poached egg and with the pitta.

Alternatively, you could transfer the pepper mixture into a microwaveproof or ovenproof dish, break the egg on top and cook in the oven for 10 minutes or so, or in the microwave for 90 seconds or so, until the egg white is cooked but the yolk still soft. This will add to the length of cooking time.

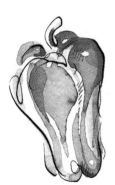 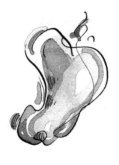

NASI GORENG

(Make-Ahead Meals, Week 5)
25 minutes to prepare and cook; will freeze

Serves 2
405 calories and 12g fat per portion

100g (dry weight) fragrant or basmati rice
1 tablespoon groundnut oil
100g lean diced chicken
1 medium carrot
4 spring onions, halved lengthways
½ teaspoon chilli flakes or sauce
1 dessertspoon light soy sauce
50g beansprouts
50g peeled prawns
1 pinch brown sugar
A little chicken stock if necessary
1 small egg

Cook the rice in water according to pack instructions; reserve.

Meanwhile, heat the oil in a non-stick frying pan and cook the chicken pieces, stirring from time to time.

Meanwhile, thinly slice the carrot lengthways, then halve and add to the cooking pan, stirring again for 2 minutes. Add the spring onions, chilli and soy sauce and stir for 2 more minutes. Add the cooked rice, beansprouts, prawns and sugar to the pan with a little chicken stock, if necessary, so it doesn't stick. Beat the egg and add it to the pan, stirring it into the rice mixture over a medium heat until cooked. Spoon the rice mixture into individual lidded freezerproof and ovenproof/microwaveproof dishes and freeze or chill. Reheat thoroughly before serving.

CASE HISTORY

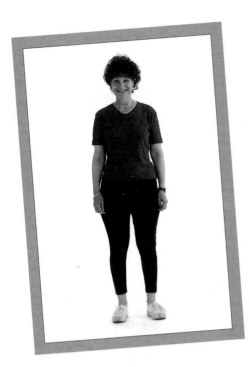

SUE RUDOLF

AGE: **53**

STATUS: **Separated for three years; two grown-up sons; lives alone**

OCCUPATION: **Press office assistant for public relations company**

HEIGHT: **5 ft 3 ins**

START WEIGHT: **9 st 7½ lb**

WEIGHT AFTER SIX WEEKS: **8 st 13 lb**

START BMI: **24.6**

BMI AFTER SIX WEEKS: **23**

START STATISTICS: **36–28–39¾**

STATISTICS AFTER SIX WEEKS: **34½–26½–38**

accepted Sue onto the programme on the condition that she realised that there was no way she would, or should, lose a stone in six weeks! There were three reasons for this: First, she was already just within the healthy BMI range of 20–25, meaning that, as explained in Chapters 1 and 2, weight loss would be slower than average. Secondly, she didn't need to lose a whole stone (though at first she told me she wanted to). For a woman, an acceptable average is a BMI of 23 – there is no need to go below that. So to reach a BMI of 23, we worked out Sue would need to lose only 8 or 9 pounds. Thirdly, Sue is a classic pear shape, with a relatively small bust and waist but large hips and thighs. This is her natural shape and, as we discussed in Chapters 1 and 2, 'pear-shaped' fat is harder to lose than 'apple-shaped' fat. Sue is also older than some of our participants and should therefore be happy with slow weight loss.

Given these factors, both Sue and I were delighted when she did, indeed, lose 8½ pounds, several inches from around her hips and thighs, and ended with a BMI of 23 precisely! Equally importantly, Sue has firmed up tremendously due to fitness consultant Sarah McClurey's exercise programme and looks amazingly different.

Says Sue, 'I've always been fairly active, and play golf every week, but my muscle tone has improved quite a lot since I started the 10-Minute tone-up. I get up earlier to do this, and go for a brisk walk several times a week. Sometimes it is hard to find the willpower, but the exercise programme is the only one I can sensibly follow considering my finances and my working life. In fact now, if I don't do the exercise, I miss it. My deportment has improved, and I feel more lithe.

'I'm delighted with the new shape of my thighs; I also hated my tummy which stuck out, but has now definitely improved. I am over the moon that I can now get in my 20-year-old Pepe jeans (in the photo!) and at last I'm confident enough to wear shorter skirts, which I've never done before.'

Sue followed the Healthy Fast Food Plan, which fitted in well with her busy, single life. 'I thought the programme was user-friendly and extremely simple to follow. It wasn't unreasonable or untenable – in fact, I really love this diet! My friends enjoyed the food when they came round, too. I'm not a saint – but then, I didn't have to be! Judith taught me lots of little gems like the one that Anchor aerosol cream is only 25 calories or so a portion – wonderful!

'I applied to join the programme after years battling with my weight, because I felt that it was probably my last chance – if I didn't get into decent shape now, I never would again in my life. Being on my own, I've got to maintain an acceptable figure in case a man might take an interest anyway!' jokes Sue. 'I feel that I look as though I've lost a stone because of being toned up. I really wouldn't have wanted to lose any more though because at my age too much weight loss can go to your face.

'It's such a relief after all these years to find a diet and fitness regime which really works!'

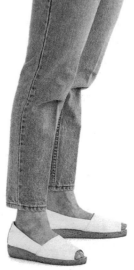

T-shirt, Pepe jeans and shoes Sue's own

the sweet-tooth plan

You want to lose weight. But you have a sweet tooth. You can't live without chocolate, or your daily biscuit fix or your regular cream cake treat – and you don't want to try.

So you don't bother trying to lose weight. It's impossible.

Well, I think you are wrong. You can slim down and still have a daily fix of sweet food; you can even have chocolate bars and those cream cakes on a regular basis.

The trick is to keep your body and your mind happy on amounts of these items which will still have you losing weight. The trick is also to get rid of the guilt that so often accompanies a sweet tooth. This chapter is all about showing you how to do these things.

Why do we have a sweet tooth?

It is often said that a sweet tooth is inborn, and that could be the case. Breast milk is sweet, which could be one reason why most children enjoy sweets and sweet foods, and why many never grow out of this.

Breast milk is also fatty. One of our main sweet-tooth addictions is for another sweet and fatty item – chocolate. And this could explain at least partly why chocolate is our number one food addiction. Chocolate is also rich in caffeine, a stimulant, phenylethylamine, a hormone linked to arousal, and theobromine, another stimulant. No wonder that chocolate has been estimated as being the downfall of around 60 per cent of all slimming diets!

Other reasons that so many of us love sweet foods are that they are easy to eat and they are instant gratification. And one scientific reason is that most sweet foods create an almost immediate increase in blood sugar levels – a sugar craving can be caused by low blood sugar and the physical feeling that you 'need something sweet'.

Are sweet foods really that bad?

The World Health Organisation recently confirmed that sugar and sweet foods **ARE HEALTHY** in moderation – up to 10 per cent of our daily calories can come from sugars. On a slimming diet such as in this chapter that means you could have 130 calories' worth, or nearly 35 grams of sugar a day. But as we have seen, sweet foods are almost always (with the exception of some confectionery and ice lollies) high or quite high in fat. It is the fat content of these items that, in the minds of most nutritionists, gives most cause for concern, as the fat in sweet foods is often saturated (the kind linked with heart disease) and a high-fat diet is also linked with weight gain and many other problems.

The World Health Organisation sets a reasonable target for daily fat intake of 30 per cent of total calories. On the slimming diet in this chapter that would represent 390 calories' worth of fat, or 43g of fat. A target of 10 per cent of total calories maximum in the form of saturated fat is reasonable, so on this diet, you can have 130 calories' worth of saturated fat a day, or 14.5g.

So how can I eat sweet/fatty foods on your diet?

What I have done is give you a weekly 'sweet treats' guideline of 1,400 calories (or an average of 200 calories a day) for sweet/fatty foods. As below, you will see you can have up to four sweet snacks a day on such a plan, so it is quite a generous allowance.

I have done this by making absolutely sure that the rest of your day's diet – a breakfast, lunch, evening meal, milk allowance and snack – is low in fat and sugar. Breakfasts contain 4g of fat or less; lunches 8g of fat or less; evening meals 12g of fat or less; your milk is virtually fat-free and your snack 2g of fat or less. This all adds up to a maximum of 26g fat a day, leaving you with 17g fat a day to 'spend' on sweet treats. I have also pared down the saturated fat in the daily meals to the minimum so that much of the 17g fat for your treat can be in the form of saturated fat.

Your daily sugar maximum allowance of 35g is more than enough to cover any sweet treat you're likely to eat. So that is how it is done!

Eating 'treat' foods is fine – as long as you keep your overall diet in balance and keep in mind my four easy steps to being boss of your own sweet tooth.

Four Easy Steps to Sweet-tooth Success

Keep your body happy

To help prevent low blood sugar you need to feed your body frequently, which is why my plan offers three meals and one healthy snack a day as well as your sweet treats. Never go more than four hours without a meal or snack while you slim. Your ideal eating pattern on this diet may be breakfast between 8 and 9am; lunch between 12 and 1pm, healthy snack about 4–4.30pm, and evening meal about 7–8pm (although if you have particular 'danger times' – see below – you may want to adjust these). In between meals you can snack on any of the 'unlimited' items (see page 73) and you also have your daily sweet treats **BUT** it is important **NOT** to eat high-sugar sweet treats when you feel very hungry and haven't eaten for a while. If you do, you may well find you eat much more than you'd planned. Try to eat your sweet treats either with a meal or snack, or soon after a meal or snack. That way you will find it much easier to eat no more than you had planned and you won't overstep your weekly allowance.

The meals and snacks within the Sweet-tooth Plan also have one other advantage – they are high in foods which take a long time to be absorbed into the bloodstream and which will keep you feeling full for longer, and keep your blood sugar levels on a more even keel.

It is important to eat everything you are allowed on the plan. Don't skip.

Some of you will have been eating much more sweet/fatty foods than you are allowed on this plan. If you eat as explained above, spacing meals out well, you shouldn't find this a problem, but if you get sweet cravings **DON'T** snack on high-calorie chocolate bars (outside your weekly allowance) but have an extra Healthy Snack, an apple, an orange, or a little dried fruit.

As explained above, when you eat high-sugar foods in between meals, your blood sugar levels tend to fluctuate, possibly causing you to crave the very foods you should be avoiding.

Keep your mind happy

You need to get your head right if you are going to follow this plan happily for the next six weeks. That means admitting that you aren't going to die if you get less than your usual amount of sweets or chocolates. It means admitting that you need to pay more attention to what you are putting in your mouth. And it means becoming a bit of a detective in spotting likely times and situations when you would normally have something sweet and fattening without even thinking about it – and lining up an alternative strategy.

I would like you to keep a diary for a week of what you eat, and every time you eat something sweet, write down why. A pattern will emerge of your danger times – both hungry times of day and times when you're eating for reasons other than hunger (of which there will be many).

Adjust your daily mealtimes to ensure that your hungriest times of day are catered for, and think up at least 10 strategies or alternatives to pigging out on sweet foods when you need comfort, when you're bored, or whatever your own danger moments are. These should be simple, immediate and non-expensive things like taking a bath, phoning a friend, going for a walk, watching a favourite video and so on.

Don't forget that eating to slim begins in the shop. What you don't buy you can't eat – so when possible plan all your meals and your sweet treats for the week, buying only what you need. If you have a family and they eat a lot of sweet food too, they could do worse than cut down with you, so if they moan because the cake tin isn't laden, for instance, tell them they will have to buy and eat their sweet foods outside the home in future!

Get rid of the guilt

The art of eating is to enjoy every last mouthful. You can't do that if you're riddled with guilt about it. So don't forget that on this plan your sweet foods are allowed, are included within your diet, are there to be savoured with not a shred of guilt at all.

Every day, plan when you are going to have your sweet treats, look forward to this and tell yourself you deserve it. This is the good way to think. If you feel guilty, there's no point.

This is especially important for anyone who has been on the binge/starve pattern. You start a diet, giving up all your favourite foods, but after a few days (or whatever) you get a massive urge to binge, do so, then feel guilty and either give up all thoughts of slimming (if you're very overweight, bad), or feel guilty and try to starve yourself (worse).

If for now you think of sweet foods as something to be enjoyed, maybe before long you will be able to think of chocolate, or whatever your treat is, as a regular part of your diet. A food that is no more important or less important than potatoes or meat or bread or milk. It's just part of your varied healthy eating plan. In other words, you like it, it's there, but it's not worth losing sleep over.

When you can get to that stage, you are in control of your sweet tooth; it isn't controlling you.

Get a life

I don't mean to be rude but sweet foods aren't the be-all and end-all of life.

I have written this plan because I would rather you lose weight with sweet foods than stay fat with sweet foods. And, at the moment, you feel there is no option.

But in the long term, sweets and cakes and chocolates aren't what you need for a happy life. Your body doesn't actually need them at all. It needs a balanced healthy diet which may include a caramel bar or a cream doughnut – but it may not.

A strange thing may happen along the way when you follow this plan. You may come to agree with me, and realise that you can go for a day or two, or more, without a sweet fix. Partly this will be because you're eating an overall more healthy, regular, varied and balanced diet. And partly this will be because your food diary and your own thoughts are making you realise that sweet treats have been taking the place of other, better things in life – like exercise, activity, fun, fashion, achievement, friends, new plans or even regular time to yourself.

Or they have been taking the place of action and therapy to sort out life's problems, such as relationship difficulties, work stress or lack of confidence. When people have problems in life, they don't turn to cabbage or skimmed milk, they turn to sweet foods. In other words, the last step to controlling your sweet food need is to begin to change not just your diet, but your life. Start making some plans now.

What to do

Read this page before beginning the plan.

Unlimiteds

Every day on the diet you can have the following items in addition to what is listed within the meals:

- *Drinks* Water, mineral water, diet fizzy drinks, low-calorie squashes, tea or coffee (black or with milk from allowance and with artificial sweetener – or sugar as part of daily treat, see below), herb teas, unsweetened fruit teas.

- *Foods* Salad vegetables, leafy green vegetables.
- *Condiments* Fresh or dried herbs and spices, lemon juice, lime juice, Worcestershire sauce, light soy sauce, tomato purée, passata, vinegar, oil-free dressings.

Milk Allowance

Every day you have an allowance of 250ml skimmed milk or 200ml semi-skimmed milk for use in tea or coffee or as a drink on its own. If not required, have one 125ml pot natural low-fat yogurt instead for the calcium content. Milk for breakfast cereals is on top of this allowance.

Meals and Snacks

The six-week plan has a week to a page. Every day during the six weeks, pick one Breakfast, one Lunch, one Evening Meal and one Healthy Snack from the options given each week.

Sweet Treats

Every week you have an allowance of 1,400 calories 'spare' so that you can choose whatever sweet treats you like to that value. This should preferably be used as 200 calories a day, certainly for the first two weeks of the plan. On pages 74–5 are my Top 40 selections for you to choose from; these vary in calories from 50 through to 200 so you can decide how you want to use your allowance – e.g. 4 × 50 calorie treats a day; 2 × 50 plus 1 × 100 calorie treats a day; 2 × 100 calorie treats a day; 1 × 50 and 1 × 150 calorie treats a day, or 1 × 200 calorie treat a day. It is up to you.

You could instead choose from the 'under 150' or 'under 200' calorie sweet recipes on pages 88–91, or you could turn to page 93 for more branded sweet foods information, or consult the nutrition tables on pages 182–8 for even more choice. If you fancy something savoury, or a glass of wine or beer, or a knob of butter, or whatever, instead – feel free to have it instead of something sweet, as long as you are sure of the exact calorie count. As long as your extras add up to no more than 200 a day, you will still lose weight.

Many branded desserts and yogurts, and other foods, give calorie information on their packs so you aren't just limited to what you can find in this book.

In the later weeks of the diet plan, you can be more flexible with your 1,400 calories a week without the need to divide this up into 200 calories a day. For instance, you might decide to have 4 × 300 calorie treats on four days plus 2 × 100 calorie treats on two days, or whatever. This will mean you can include any of the higher-calorie recipe dishes on pages 91–2, and more of the items listed on page 93. But using the whole 1,400 calories up in one day isn't advisable – try to spread it out.

Eat sweet treats with, or soon after, a meal. Remember – don't feel guilty; this allowance forms a legitimate part of your overall healthy slimming plan.

Fill out the diary. Every week there is space for you to fill in your sweet treats so that there is no chance of you forgetting what you've had. Do fill it in – it will help.

Men

Have 1/3 larger portions of potatoes, bread, rice, pasta, etc. and as much extra milk as you like.

40 Sweet Snacks You Can Enjoy Without Guilt

Use these snacks as part of your Sweet-tooth Plan, the instructions for which appear on the previous page.

50 calories or less

- 1 dark rye Ryvita spread generously with chocolate spread, any variety.
- 1 Rich Tea biscuit spread with Provender low-fat dark chocolate spread.
- 1 sachet instant low-fat hot chocolate drink, any variety, made up.
- Up to 1 whole sachet sugar-free jelly (up to a pint).
- 1 Yoplait Frubes 40g tube.
- 3 rounded teaspoonfuls sugar (for use in tea or coffee).

100 calories or less

- 1 × 2-pack Weight Watchers cookies, any variety.
- 1 Go Ahead Caramel Crisp bar.
- 1 Prewett's Carob Fruit and Nut bar.
- 1 Quaker Harvest Choc Chip Chewy bar.
- 1 round crumpet generously spread with low-sugar jam.
- 1 Lo bar (not Gold), orange or mint flavour.
- 2 fingers KitKat.
- 1 Cadbury's Dairy Milk Mousse.
- 1 individual pot Ambrosia low-fat Devon custard.
- 1 Lyons Maid Mivvi, any flavour.
- 1 individual tub Wall's Blue Ribbon ice cream.
- 1 Häagen-Dazs Frozen Yogurt bar, any flavour

150 calories or less

- 1 Hob Nob individual bar.
- 1 Shepherdboy Apple Fruit and Nut bar.
- 1 Cadbury's Caramel cake bar.
- 1 Mr Kipling Almond Slice.
- 1 Lyons Cup Cake, any variety.
- 1 Lyons Jam Tart.
- 1 individual pot Ambrosia Creamed Rice or custard (full fat).
- 1 Boots Shapers Blackcurrant Cheesecake.
- 1 Cadbury's Turkish Delight Dessert.
- 1 Aero Mousse.

200 calories or less

- 1 Mars Tracker Choc Chip.
- 1 Rowntree's Chunky Aero bar.
- 1 Rowntree's medium Golden Cup bar.
- 1 Cadbury's Crunchie bar.
- 1 Cadbury's Creme Egg.
- 1 Cadbury's Wispa bar.
- 1 Nestle's Milky Bar, chunky.
- 1 Mr Kipling Strawberry Sundae or Cherry Bakewell.
- 1 individual Weight Watchers Chocolate Sensations cheesecake.
- 1 Cadbury's Caramel ice cream.
- 1 Cadbury's Dairy Milk choc ice.
- 1 Wall's Strawberry Cornetto.

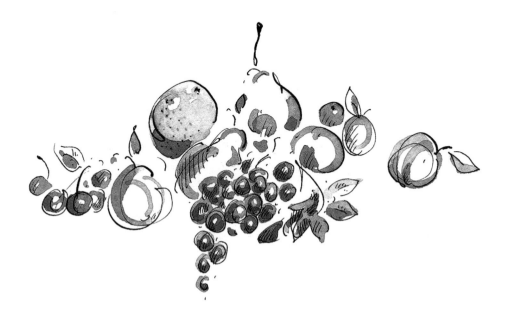

WEEK ONE

Notes

- Don't forget your 'Unlimiteds' and Sweet Treats (see page 73).
- Unless otherwise stated, bread is 1 slice of brown, white or wholemeal bread from a large, medium-cut sliced loaf and it is very lightly spread with low-fat spread.
- Try to vary your meal choices as much as possible.

Breakfasts

- 25g All-Bran with 125ml skimmed milk and 1 medium banana.
- 1 slice bread or toast with low-sugar jam or marmalade; 1 Shape diet fruit yogurt; 1 plum, nectarine or satsuma.
- 25g cornflakes with 125ml skimmed milk and 40g ready-to-eat dried apricots (5 apricot pieces), chopped in.

Lunches

- Sandwich of 2 slices bread filled with 40g low-fat soft cheese and salad; 1 apple.
- Bowl New Covent Garden Minestrone or Heinz Thick Country Vegetable with Ham soup; 1 slice bread; 1 kiwifruit or satsuma.
- 1 small wholemeal roll with a very little low-fat spread; 1 medium cooked chicken breast portion, skin removed; fresh salad selection with oil-free French dressing or balsamic vinegar; medium slice melon or 1 plum.
- 200g baked beans on 1 slice toast; 1 orange or 2 satsumas.

Evening Meals

- 50g (dry weight) pasta cooked and topped with 4 tablespoons ready-made Italian Tomato Sauce plus 1 tablespoon grated Parmesan cheese; large side salad; small apple.
- 200g white fish steak or fillet, grilled, microwaved or baked; 150g new or boiled potatoes; 3 tablespoons peas; 1 level dessertspoon tomato sauce or Free Choice mayonnaise; 1 medium banana.
- 1 × 150g turkey fillet, sliced and stir-fried with a selection of thinly sliced fresh vegetables in 1 dessertspoon oil with light soy sauce and 1 level dessertspoon Sharwood's Hoi Sin Sauce and chicken stock as necessary; 3 tablespoons cooked rice.
- 1 portion Tarragon Pork (see recipe page 63).
- 1 pack Findus Lean Cuisine Premium Chicken à l'Orange; 1 apple.

Healthy Snacks

- 1 large banana.
- 5 ready-to-eat stoned prunes; 1 apple.
- 15g shelled sunflower seeds.
- 125g pot Danone Bio Yogurt Lite, any flavour.

Sweet Treats Record

	Had	Calories	Running total
Monday	_____	_____	_____
Tuesday	_____	_____	_____
Wednesday	_____	_____	_____
Thursday	_____	_____	_____
Friday	_____	_____	_____
Saturday	_____	_____	_____
Sunday	_____	_____	_____
Week Total			1,400 calories

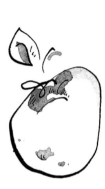
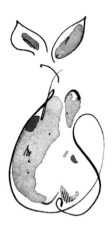

WEEK TWO

Notes

- Try to space your meals out evenly.
- Remember to eat Sweet Treats with or shortly after a meal or snack.

Breakfasts

- 1 large banana; 1 × 200g pot Müller Light banana or vanilla yogurt.
- 1 Nutri-Grain morning bar, blueberry or strawberry; 1 Shape diet fromage frais.
- 1 slice toast, with Marmite; 25g All-Bran with milk from allowance; 1 plum, satsuma or kiwi fruit.

Lunches

- Sandwich of 2 slices bread filled with 1 medium hard-boiled egg, 1 teaspoon Free Choice mayonnaise and salad; 1 apple.
- 1 × 425g can Baxters Chilli Bean Hotpot soup; 1 mini pitta; kiwi fruit.
- 1 pack Weight Watchers Vegetable Balti with Naan Bread (chilled); salad.
- 1 × 85g pot Iceland 95 per cent fat free BBQ dip with selection of vegetable crudités plus 2 Sunblest Wholewheat Crisprolls; 1 Shape Twinpot bio yogurt, strawberry flavour.

Evening Meals

- 1 × 225g baked potato; 1 medium chicken breast portion, baked in foil with lemon juice, herbs and seasoning; 3 tablespoons sweetcorn, 1 portion 'unlimited' leafy greens.
- Tuna and Vegetable Stir-fry (see recipe page 60).
- Chicken Satay (see recipe page 152).
- 1 Weight Watchers 400g Tagliatelle Carbonara; large mixed salad.
- Macaroni cheese made (for one portion) with 50g macaroni, cooked and mixed with quarter pack Napolina Creamy Bake Lasagne Sauce plus 75g cooked broccoli florets and garnished with 1 sliced tomato and 25g grated half-fat mozzarella cheese. (If serving more, simply multiply the ingredients accordingly.)

Healthy Snacks

- 1 slice of bread with pure fruit spread.
- 1 Shape Bio Twinpot, plum and blackcurrant flavour.
- 1 mini pitta filled with salad items and oil-free French dressing or balsamic vinegar.

Sweet Treats Record

	Had	Calories	Running total
Monday			
Tuesday			
Wednesday			
Thursday			
Friday			
Saturday			
Sunday			
Week Total			1,400 calories

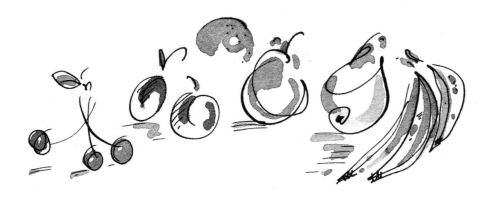

WEEK **THREE**

Notes

- Don't forget to include plenty of 'unlimited' vegetables with your evening meals and salad stuff with your lunches.
- You can choose meals from other weeks in the programme to vary your diet more, as long as you pick one Breakfast, one Lunch, one Evening Meal and one Healthy Snack a day.

Breakfasts

- 2–3 large tomatoes, quartered and grilled or dry-fried in a non-stick pan with Fry Light spray, served on 1½ slices toast; with 1 level tablespoon grated Parmesan cheese sprinkled over.
- 40g no added sugar or salt muesli with 100ml skimmed milk and ½ pink grapefruit.
- 25g branflakes with 140ml skimmed milk; 1 medium banana.

Lunches

- Sandwich of 2 slices bread filled with 60g peeled prawns and salad; 1 Shape fruit-on-the-bottom fromage frais, any flavour.
- 1 white large pitta bread split and filled with 50g hummus and a variety of chopped firm salad items such as cucumber, peppers, celery, onion, tomato. Lettuce and cress can be added if eating straight away.
- 1 x 450ml pack St Michael Tomato and Basil soup sprinkled with 1 rounded tablespoon grated half-fat mozzarella cheese, 1 Weight Watchers soft brown roll or 1 slice bread.
- 1 Boots Shapers tuna and cucumber sandwich; 1 large banana.

Evening Meals

- ½ a 283g can ratatouille heated and mixed with 50g (dry weight) pasta shapes, cooked, and topped with 1 tablespoon grated Parmesan cheese; salad.
- 1 portion Penne Primavera (see recipe page 66).
- 1 portion Sweet and Sour Pork with Noodles (see recipe page 64).
- 1 medium rainbow trout (250g), cooked without fat; 125g new or boiled potatoes; 4 tablespoons peas; unlimited greens; horseradish sauce.
- Omelette made with 2 medium eggs cooked in a non-stick pan sprayed with Fry Light, filled with chopped mushrooms; 1 small wholemeal roll; salad; 1 Müller Light 200g pot fruit yogurt.

Healthy Snacks

- 1 rounded tablespoon hummus on 1 dark rye Ryvita.
- 5 dried ready-to-eat apricots plus one apple.
- 40g tzatziki (yogurt and cucumber) with raw carrot or other vegetable plus one Grissini stick.

Sweet Treats Record

	Had	Calories	Running total
Monday	_____	_____	_____
Tuesday	_____	_____	_____
Wednesday	_____	_____	_____
Thursday	_____	_____	_____
Friday	_____	_____	_____
Saturday	_____	_____	_____
Sunday	_____	_____	_____
Week Total			1,400 calories

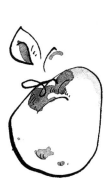
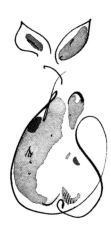

WEEK **FOUR**

Notes

- Don't forget to drink plenty of fluids on the plan – water is the best drink of all! Low-calorie squashes and fizzy drinks may help appease your sweet tooth in the short term but long term it is a good idea to try to limit them as they contain lots of unnatural additives.

Breakfasts

- 125ml natural low-fat bio yogurt topped with medium portion chopped fruit or berry fruits, 1 teaspoon caster sugar, and 1 small handful All-Bran.
- 2 Weetabix with 125ml skimmed milk; ½ pink grapefruit.
- 1 slice bread with low-sugar jam or marmalade; 1 Shape fromage frais; 1 apple.
- 5 tablespoons baked beans on 1 slice toast; ½ pink grapefruit.

Lunches

- 75g French bread; 30g reduced-fat farmhouse Cheddar, 1 teaspoon pickle, tomato and onion salad with oil-free French dressing.
- 1 × 100g can tuna in water or brine, drained, flaked and tossed with 50g (canned, drained) butter beans, 1 large sliced tomato, 3 chopped spring onions and oil-free French dressing; 1 slice bread.

- 1 carton New Covent Garden Tuscan Bean soup; 2 Sunblest Cracked Wheat Crisprolls.
- Rice salad: mix 6 tablespoons cooked rice (preferably brown) with ½ chopped red apple, 3 chopped dried ready-to-eat apricots, 50g chopped cooked lean chicken, and unlimited chopped salad items, tossed in oil-free French dressing; 1 medium banana.

Evening Meals

- Moroccan Lamb with Couscous (see recipe page 65).
- Jambalaya (see recipe page 157).
- 100g salmon fillet or steak, cooked without fat; 125g new or boiled potatoes; medium portion green beans and broccoli; 1 apple.
- Aubergine and Lentil Curry (see recipe page 111).
- 1 × 250g baked potato topped with 4 tablespoons baked beans and 25g half-fat grated mozzarella cheese; salad.

Healthy Snacks

- 1 large banana.
- 15g pumpkin seeds.
- 1 Shape fromage frais and 1 satsuma.
- 2 dark rye Ryvitas with Marmite.

Sweet Treats Record

	Had	Calories	Running total
Monday			
Tuesday			
Wednesday			
Thursday			
Friday			
Saturday			
Sunday			
Week Total			1,400 calories

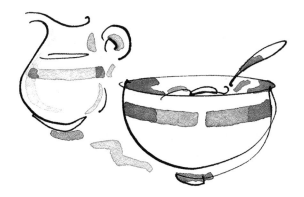

WEEK FIVE

Notes

Don't forget the delicious sweet recipes on pages 88–91. They are all quick and easy to do.

Breakfasts

- 1 wholemeal English muffin with low-fat spread and a little low-sugar jam; ½ grapefruit.
- 25g All-Bran with 125ml skimmed milk; 1 medium chopped banana.
- 1 Weetabix with milk from allowance; ½ grapefruit; 1 slice bread with low-sugar jam or marmalade.

Lunches

- Sandwich of 2 slices bread filled with 50g wafer-thin turkey and salad with 1 teaspoon Free Choice mayonnaise; 1 pear or 1 Shape fruit yogurt.
- 1 can Weight Watchers Mediterranean Tomato and Red Pepper soup; 1 wholemeal bap filled with 1 medium egg, hard-boiled and sliced, and salad with 1 teaspoon Free Choice mayonnaise or low-fat Thousand Island dressing.
- Pasta salad: mix 50g (dry weight) pasta shapes, cooked, with 25g crumbled feta cheese, 1 ripe fresh chopped tomato, chopped cucumber, celery and sweet pepper, all tossed in oil-free French dressing.
- Large mixed salad with oil-free dressing or 1 dessertspoonful Free Choice mayonnaise, with 3 slices extra lean ham from a vacuum pack (75g); 1 wholemeal bap with a little low-fat spread; 1 apple.

Evening Meals

- Roast chicken dinner: 110g lean roast chicken meat (about three slices); 2 small chunks roast potato or 1 large (80g); 3 tablespoons peas or sweetcorn; unlimited leafy vegetables, portion carrots; gravy skimmed of fat; 1 low-fat chipolata sausage, baked, or 1 dessertspoon stuffing.
- 1 portion Turkey and Mushroom Filo Pie (see recipe page 153); 3 tablespoons instant mashed potato or potato boiled and mashed with a little skimmed milk; unlimited leafy greens.
- 200g cod, cooked without fat; 125g Beefeater (thick cut) oven chips; 3 tablespoons peas.
- 1 × 285g St Michael 95 per cent Fat Free Stonebake Vegetable Pizza; large salad.
- 175g grilled beef steak; with 175g new potatoes; 4 tablespoons peas or sweetcorn or large mixed salad with oil-free French dressing or 1 dessertspoon Free Choice mayonnaise.
- 1 Weight Watchers Vegetable Lasagne; salad; large banana.

Healthy Snacks

- 1 apple, 1 orange.
- 15g sunflower seeds.
- 1 Shape diet fromage frais, 1 satsuma.

Sweet Treats Record

	Had	Calories	Running total
Monday	_____	_____	_____
Tuesday	_____	_____	_____
Wednesday	_____	_____	_____
Thursday	_____	_____	_____
Friday	_____	_____	_____
Saturday	_____	_____	_____
Sunday	_____	_____	_____
Week Total			1,400 calories

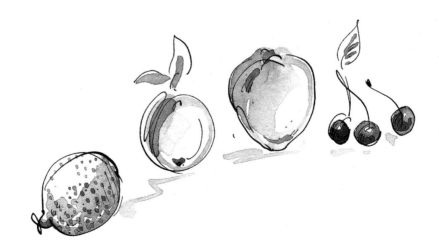

WEEK SIX

Notes

- Are you eating plenty of fruit and vegetables? You should aim for five portions a day.
- When you have finished Week 6, turn to Chapter 10 for what to do next.

Breakfasts

- 125g tub natural low-fat bio yogurt topped with 125g stewed apple, sweetened with a little fructose and 10g (small handful) All-Bran.
- Müller Light yogurt, any variety; 1 large banana.
- ½ pink grapefruit; 1 Shape diet yogurt; 1 slice bread with low-sugar jam or marmalade.

Lunches

- Sandwich of 2 slices bread filled with 50g smoked salmon and sliced cucumber; 75g grapes or cherries.
- Crab salad: 1 average dressed crab with plenty of unlimited salad items and 1 level tablespoon Free Choice mayonnaise; 1 wholemeal bap with a little low-fat spread.
- 1 x 405g can Heinz Thick Country Vegetable Soup with Ham with 1 dessertspoon Parmesan cheese grated over plus 1 slice bread; 1 plum or satsuma.
- 1 medium egg, poached, on 1 slice toast; 1 Shape diet fromage frais; 1 orange.
- 1 Boots Shapers Lemon Chicken or Prawn Cocktail sandwich; 1 apple.

Evening Meals

- 1 portion Chilli Con Carne (see recipe page 154); 5 tablespoons of plain boiled rice; side salad.
- Pork kebabs: thread 175g lean pork fillet, cubed, onto a skewer, brush with a little olive oil and grill, turning once, for 10 minutes, then sprinkle with a little salt and plenty of lemon juice; large salad dressed with a little olive oil; 4 tablespoons cooked rice.
- 1 portion Quick Pasta Gratin (see recipe page 106); salad or green beans.
- 50g (dry weight) spaghetti, cooked and topped with ½ 250g jar Napolina Tomato, Salmon and Mascarpone Sauce, 1 tablespoon grated Parmesan cheese; large side salad; 1 apple.
- 1 Quorn Balti Jalfrezi with Naan Bread; tomato and onion side salad.

Healthy Snacks

- Quarter portion Tuna Pâté (see recipe page 60) on 1 dark rye Ryvita.
- 2 rice cakes topped with 30g low-fat soft cheese and apple slices.
- 5 ready-to-eat dried stoned prunes and 1 Shape diet fromage frais.

Sweet Treats Record

	Had	Calories	Running total
Monday	_____	_____	_____
Tuesday	_____	_____	_____
Wednesday	_____	_____	_____
Thursday	_____	_____	_____
Friday	_____	_____	_____
Saturday	_____	_____	_____
Sunday	_____	_____	_____
Week Total			1,400 calories

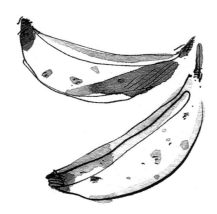

SWEET-TOOTH RECIPES

150 CALORIES OR UNDER

CHOCOLATE PEARS

Serves 4
150 calories and 2.5g fat per portion

4 nice large pears – e.g. William or Conference
Lemon juice
50ml golden syrup
2 level tablespoons cocoa powder
4 scoops Weight Watchers Chocolate Swirl ice cream

Peel the pears leaving stalks in place, cut off bottoms to make a flat base, brush with lemon juice and put upright in a small saucepan in about 2cm of water. Bring to a simmer, cover and cook gently until tender.

Meanwhile, heat the syrup in a small pan and stir in the cocoa, mixing until you have a smooth sauce. When the pears are cooked, remove from the pan with a slotted spoon and serve with the sauce poured over and a scoop of ice cream on each.

CHOCOLATE AND STRAWBERRY MERINGUES

Serves 4
150 calories and 2.5g fat per portion

2 × 125g tubs Puddi chocolate puddings
4 ready-made meringue nests
100g strawberries
1 level dessertspoon icing sugar
4 good squirts of Anchor aerosol cream, any flavour

Spoon half a chocolate pudding into each of the meringue nests. Slice the strawberries and fill each nest, then dust with icing sugar. Top each with a good squirt of aerosol cream and serve immediately.

NOTE *You could use raspberries or stoned halved cherries in this recipe instead of strawberries.*

BLACK FOREST DESSERT

Serves 4
150 calories and 5g fat per portion

290g can black cherries in juice
1 teaspoon arrowroot powder
1 sachet instant hot chocolate drink
100g 8 per cent fat fromage frais
4 × 68g tubs Weight Watchers Chocolate Mousse

Drain the cherries, reserving the juice. Heat the juice in a pan with the arrowroot until you have a thickened sauce. In a mug or small heatproof bowl, mix the sachet of hot chocolate with enough boiling water to make a smooth chocolate sauce the consistency of single cream, then mix the sauce into the fromage frais. Dividing the cherries, cherry sauce, fromage frais and mousses evenly between four glass dishes or glasses, make each dessert as follows: spoon half the cherries into the dishes; spoon the fromage frais/chocolate sauce in next, then the chocolate mousse and finally the rest of the cherries topped with the cherry sauce.

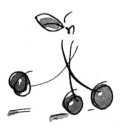

CHOCOLATE BROWNIES

Makes 12
120 calories and 4.5g fat each

Fry Light spray
175g Go Ahead Golden Crunch biscuits
75g Rice Krispies
75g half-fat Anchor spread
50ml golden syrup
4 × 68g tubs Weight Watchers Chocolate Mousse

Spray a square non-stick baking tin with the Fry Light spray. Crush the biscuits between kitchen parchment with a rolling pin and mix with the Rice Krispies. Melt the half-fat spread and syrup in a small pan and mix into the biscuit mixture. Stir in the mousses and mix everything together well, then smooth into the baking tin and allow to set in the refrigerator for a few hours before cutting into 12 pieces.

BAKED BANANAS WITH CHOCOLATE SAUCE

Serves 4
132 calories and 1g fat per portion

4 medium bananas
50ml golden syrup
2 level tablespoons cocoa powder

Bake the bananas in their skins in the oven at 180°C/350°F/Gas 4 for 20 minutes or until the skins are blackened.

Meanwhile, heat the syrup in a small saucepan and stir in the cocoa powder until you have a smooth sauce. When the bananas are cooked, serve each on a plate, slit lengthways down the top with the sauce poured into the open skin.

200 CALORIES OR UNDER

PASSION CAKE SLICES

175 calories and 7.5g fat per slice

Fry Light spray
200g plain or wholemeal flour
1 teaspoon baking powder
1 pinch ground cinnamon and ginger
50g half-fat Anchor spread
50g golden caster sugar
1 medium fresh carrot, peeled and grated
60g chopped mixed nuts
4 level tablespoons lemon curd
50ml skimmed milk
1 medium egg
1 × 350g tub 8 per cent fat fromage frais
1 tablespoon icing sugar
1 tablespoon lemon juice

Spray a non-stick oblong baking tin with Fry Light. In a mixing bowl, combine the flour, baking powder and spices. Rub in the half-fat spread, then add the sugar, carrot and mixed nuts. In a small bowl, mix together the lemon curd, skimmed milk and egg until well combined, and add to the flour mixture, stirring well. Spoon into the baking tin and level the surface. Bake at 180°C/350°F/Gas 4 for 30 minutes or until a skewer comes out of the centre clean and the cake looks golden. Turn out and allow to cool.

Meanwhile, make a topping by beating the fromage frais with the icing sugar and lemon juice. Spread over the cake when cool, then cut into 12 slices. The top can be decorated with slices of lemon or walnut halves (20 calories and 2g fat each).

COFFEE, TOFFEE AND CHOCOLATE DELIGHTS

Serves 4
175 calories and 7.2g fat per portion

8 sponge fingers

6 tablespoons strong coffee

3 × 150g Shape low-fat toffee yogurts

2 tablespoons Smuckers Light Hot Chocolate Fudge
   Topping

1 Flake treatsize bar

Use four glass dishes or glasses. Break the sponge fingers in half and place four halves in each glass. Pour the coffee evenly over them. Spoon three-quarters of a tub of yogurt into each, heat the topping and drizzle a quarter over each dessert, then sprinkle each with a quarter of the Flake bar, crumbled.

ORANGE LIQUEUR FRUIT TRIFLE

Serves 4
200 calories and 3.5g fat per portion

3 trifle sponge cakes, each halved horizontally

1 dessertspoon raspberry jam

175ml orange juice

1 tablespoon orange liqueur, e.g. Grand Marnier

2 small bananas

1 × 290g can Birds low-fat custard

8 squirts aerosol cream

Spread the sponges with the jam, put the halved slices back together again and cut each sponge cake into four. Put three sponge pieces in the base of each of four individual trifle dishes. Mix the orange juice with the liqueur and pour evenly over the sponges. Slice the banana and divide between the dishes, then top immediately with the custard and finish with 2 squirts of aerosol cream each.

PEAR AND CHOCOLATE HONEY CREAMS

Serves 4
200 calories and 4.5g fat per portion

1 × 400g can pears in juice, drained

2 Halo Honey Malt chocolate bars

100g 8 per cent fat fromage frais

100g half-fat crème fraîche

2 × 200g pots Müller Light vanilla yogurt

1 level tablespoon runny honey

Chop the pears and place in four individual glass dishes or glasses. Chop the Halo bars and spoon half over the pears. Blend together the fromage frais and crème fraîche and spoon a quarter into each dish. Spoon the vanilla yogurt over the top and finish with the rest of the chopped chocolate and a drizzle of honey on each dessert.

250 CALORIES OR UNDER

QUICK CREAMY BRÛLÉE

Serves 4
240 calories and 13.5g fat per portion

75g mascarpone cheese

200g 8 per cent fat fromage frais

200g low-fat ready-made custard

125g frozen raspberries, blackberries or other soft fruit

4 tablespoons caster sugar

Beat together the mascarpone with the fromage frais, then stir in the custard to combine well.

Meanwhile, heat the fruit in a small pan with ½ tablespoon of the sugar until the juices are just starting to run, and divide between four small heatproof ramekins. Spoon a quarter of the cheese mixture over the top of each of these and level out, then top each with a quarter of the remaining sugar. Grill under a preheated very hot grill to caramelise the sugar. Leave to cool before serving.

CHOCOLATE AND COCONUT CRUNCHIES

Serves 4
247 calories and 14.5g fat per portion

250g tub 8 per cent fat fromage frais

1 sachet low-calorie instant hot chocolate drink

30g desiccated coconut

37g pack Maltesers, crushed

6 gingernut biscuits, lightly crushed

Put the fromage frais in a mixing bowl. Blend the chocolate drink with 30ml boiling water and stir this into the fromage frais. Mix in the coconut and Maltesers. Divide the mixture between four small dishes or glasses and top with the crushed gingernut biscuits.

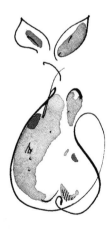

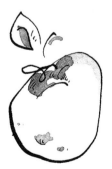

300 CALORIES OR UNDER

BANOFFEE LAYERS

Serves 4
267 calories and 8g fat per portion

2 bananas
4 individual Shape creamy toffee bio yogurts
1 large Cadbury's Caramel bar
30ml single cream
150ml thick bio yogurt
1 dessertspoon icing sugar
1 Flake treatsize bar

Slice the bananas thinly and arrange in the base of
four glass serving dishes or glasses. Spoon half a pot
of toffee yogurt into each dish. Melt the Caramel bar
in a small pan with the single cream, mix well and
divide this mixture between the four dishes. Beat the
bio yogurt with the icing sugar and spoon one
quarter into each dish. Top with the remaining toffee
yogurts and finish by crumbling the Flake and
sprinkling it over the top of the desserts.

TIRAMISU

Serves 4
260 calories and 14g fat per portion

12 sponge fingers
50ml Marsala wine
75ml strong coffee
25g fructose
75g mascarpone cheese
200g 8 per cent fat fromage frais
100ml half-fat crème fraîche
1 level tablespoon cocoa powder

Put the sponge fingers in a four-serving trifle bowl.
Mix the Marsala, coffee and fructose and pour evenly
over the sponge fingers. Beat together the cheese
and fromage frais; beat in the crème fraîche and
spoon evenly over the fingers. Top with the cocoa
powder sieved over.

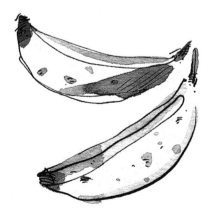

CALORIE AND FAT GUIDE to All Your Favourite Sweet-tooth Products

Use this list in conjunction with the instructions for the Sweet-tooth Plan that appear on pages 73–4. Some more basic sweet foods appear in the nutrition listings at the end of the book.

Biscuits and Snack Bars	Calories	Fat (g)
Typical values per biscuit (brands may vary slightly)		
Chocolate digestive	85	4
Chocolate finger	30	1.5
Custard cream	65	3
Digestive	80	4
Gingernut	40	1.3
Jaffa cake	45	1
Rich Tea	40	1.4
Shortcake	65	3.5
Jacob's Club milk	122	6.5
Jordan's Crunchy Bar	155	7.5
Nutri-Grain morning bar, strawberry	140	3
Quaker Harvest Chewy bars	max 100	max 3.7
Mars Tracker, choc chip, individual	196	10.7
Sunwheel Flapjack, 80g, honey/raisin	393	20.5

Ices	Calories	Fat (g)
Lyons Maid Extreme Vanilla	369	19.9
Mars (single)	209	12
Nestlé KitKat	218	14.5
Wall's Cornetto, choc'n nut	220	12
Wall's Magnum Classic	295	20

Sweets	Calories	Fat (g)
Starburst, 45g	185	3.4
Fox's Glacier Mints, one stick pack	144	nil
Fruit Gums, 1 tube	137	nil
Fruit Pastilles, 1 tube	147	nil
Polo Mints, 1 tube	120	0.3

Cakes and pastries	Calories	Fat (g)
Mr Kipling Bakewell Slice	137	6.3
Mr Kipling Bramley Apple Pie	230	8.3
Mr Kipling Luxury Mince Pie	250	9.2
Mr Kipling Mini Battenberg	126	2.8
Chocolate eclair, large (average)	260	20
Carrot cake, iced, average 75g slice	300	15
Victoria jam sponge, average 50g slice	200	11
Chocolate fudge cake, average 75g slice	290	15
Rich fruit cake, iced, average 50g slice	180	5
Coffee and walnut sponge, iced, average 50g slice	220	12
Doughnut, jam, average	250	12
Cream or vanilla slice	300	18

Chocolates	Calories	Fat (g)
Cadbury's Boost	280	16
Cadbury's Caramel	240	12
Cadbury's Crunchie treatsize	80	3.2
Cadbury's Dairy Milk, standard	255	14.5
Cadbury's Fudge	120	4.5
Fry's Chocolate Cream	215	7
Mars Bar, 65g	295	11.5
Mars Flyte	196	6.6
Mars Milky Way, twin	236	8.6
Nestlé Aero milk, medium	252	14.4
KitKat, 4 finger	244	12.6
Rolos, one tube	250	11
Yorkie, milk, 6 chunk	295	16.5
Toblerone, 32g bar	168	9.2

NOTE *Calorie and fat counts for individual chilled or frozen desserts and yogurts almost always appear on the pack. Any of them can be included in your diet as long as the calorie and fat count falls within your weekly allowance (see page 73).*

CASE HISTORY

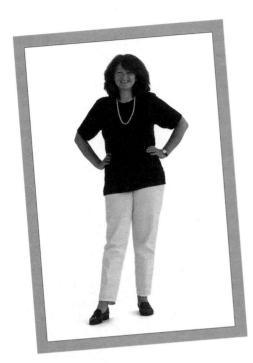

DANA MILLS

AGE: **34**
STATUS: **Married; two boys aged 4 and 5**
OCCUPATION: **Housewife**
HEIGHT: **5 ft 7½ ins**
START WEIGHT: **13 st**
WEIGHT AFTER SIX WEEKS: **12 st**
START BMI: **29.2**
BMI AFTER SIX WEEKS: **26.9**
START STATISTICS: **43¼–35–45½**
STATISTICS AFTER SIX WEEKS: **42–32–42**

Dana has always adored food and been overweight since her early twenties. The weight had gradually increased, no doubt partly due to having her two boys and also to her self-confessed sweet tooth, until her alltime high of 13 stone, giving her a BMI dangerously near to clinically obese (30+).

Dana had also recently moved to London from Devon with her family, and was finding it a bit too big and lonely, and was worried that if she didn't tackle her weight things would just get worse. 'I am a great comfort eater and always turn to sweet food during low times.

'My motivation to join the programme was that all my clothes had become too tight to wear, especially my jeans and fitted skirts. My weight was really escalating and I felt out of control.'

Dana's pre-plan food diary showed me that she had been snacking regularly throughout the day (a self-confessed 'grazer') including regular 'fixes' of sweet foods – cakes, chocolate and biscuits were three of her favourites. As she took little exercise except a visit to the swimming pool most weeks, no wonder the weight had been creeping on.

I put Dana on the Sweet-tooth Plan, splitting up her meals and snacks so that she could eat five times a day, which would help keep hunger pangs at bay. She found the reduction in calories very hard for the first few days and so we upped her calorie allowance a little (the more overweight you are, the more you can eat and still lose weight) and after that she coped very well.

'My husband was really supportive and actually did the programme alongside me, losing nearly a stone too. I tried to do as much walking and swimming as possible while on the plan, which wasn't easy with two small children. Vigorous exercise can be deeply uncomfortable if you have a big bust, so these were the two activities I felt most happy with.

'The main difference after the six weeks is how I look – I feel a whole lot better in my clothes, and so it has increased my confidence. My husband Piers loves my new shape and he loves the fact that I can wear more fitted, slightly sexier clothes. I went out with my mother at the end of the six weeks and I bought myself some new clothes to celebrate!'

The programme has motivated Dana to go on and lose another stone (which would bring her BMI just within the healthy 20–25 range) and to carry on eating more healthily. 'I will carry on with the programme to get another 14 lb off at least. I can't say my tastes in food have changed radically, but I try to eat more healthily. I do enjoy yogurt now, I eat more fruit and vegetables, I cook plenty of stir-fries with lots of vegetables and lean meat, and I love pitta bread.'

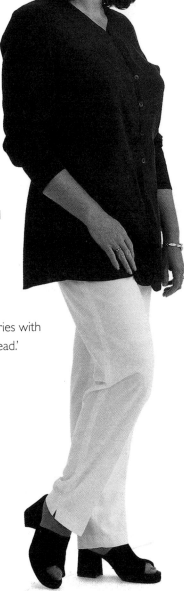

Top and trousers Dana's own, Grattan velvet mules.

the meat-free plan

The majority of us still eat meat and enjoy it – but there is an ever-growing band who don't – and an even larger one who often think they would like to try going vegetarian – or almost vegetarian – but aren't quite brave enough to take the step.

Many people give up meat and animal products for compassionate reasons. Just as many give up because they believe that a vegetarian diet will help them to health.

We now know that this certainly can be the case. Statistics show that vegetarians are less at risk from coronary heart disease and some cancers than are meat-eaters. They are also less prone to high blood pressure and strokes. Interestingly, they also, on average, weigh less than non-vegetarians.

So perhaps if you are overweight and have other risk factors for heart disease or cancer

- high blood pressure
- family history of CHD, breast or bowel cancer
- you smoke

(these and other risk factors your doctor will discuss with you) it may make sense to consider going vegetarian, or at least demi-vegetarian.

If you've ever thought of giving up meat, perhaps now is the time.

Why is a vegetarian diet so healthy?

A balanced vegetarian diet relying heavily on plant foods is:
- High in fibre from fruit, vegetables, pulses and whole grains.
- High in anti-oxidant vitamins, minerals and other plant chemicals that help protect against disease; these are found in fruits, vegetables, pulses and whole grains.
- Low in the saturated fats found in greatest quantities in meat and animal produce.

Whereas a carnivore diet is often high in saturates and low in fibre, fruit, vegetables, pulses and whole grains. In other words, a vegetarian diet fits in well with international guidelines on healthy eating and disease prevention.

Or, at least, it should.

In truth, many vegetarians still do eat a lot of saturated fat because they replace meat in the diet with an abundance of dairy produce and eggs. Full-fat dairy produce such as Cheddar cheese, full-fat milk and cream is actually higher in saturated fats than meat is. Other vegetarians may eat a very unbalanced diet, perhaps relying on sweet foods, pastries and other refined carbohydrates and still not eating enough fruit, vegetables, pulses or wholegrain cereals.

So going vegetarian doesn't guarantee that you will have a healthy diet – you still have to know what you're doing and balance it out.

The following information gives plenty of tips for new vegetarians and the diet, with some tasty recipes, shows how to build the healthy foods such as more vegetables and pulses into your regular diet while you lose weight.

A small percentage of vegetarians eat no dairy produce or other animal produce at all, and these are called vegans. Veganism is beyond the scope of this diet but it is suitable for everyone else. If you are a 'demi-veg', wishing to eat fish in your diet, I have included some fish alternatives in the six-week plan – choose them if you want to. In fact, there is an argument on health grounds for eating fish regularly even if you give up meat – all fish is low in saturated fat, white fish is very low in all fats, and fatty fish like salmon is high in special polyunsaturated fats which are part of the omega-3 group of essential fats, linked with protection against coronary artery disease and stroke.

Tips for new vegetarians

If you follow the tips here you should avoid the few problems some people complain about when switching to a vegetarian diet – digestive problems, lack of variety or taste in meals and problems fitting a vegetarian diet in with non-vegetarian members of the family. I also give tips on making sure that all the nutrients you need are included in your diet.

Acclimatise gradually

If your diet has up until now been high in meat and low in plant foods, it is wisest to let your digestive system adapt over a period of 2–3 weeks to a different way of eating. Going from a low-fibre diet to a high one overnight can result in heartburn, wind, stomach cramps and even diarrhoea.

Here is a plan to help you avoid this:

- **Week 1** Cut out red meat from your diet, replacing it with fish. Eat one extra portion of vegetables and one portion of whole grains (e.g. cereals, wholemeal bread, rather than just using refined cereals and white bread) a day.

- **Week 2** Cut out poultry, too, this week and cut down on full-fat dairy produce, replacing them with dishes based on pulses (you'll find several in the recipe section). Increase the amount of fruit that you eat to two portions a day, and eat more of your vegetables raw – in salad form. Increase whole grains again and add some nuts and seeds to your diet.

- **Week 3** Your full vegetarian diet (include 2–3 portions of fish a week if you are going demi-veg). Cut out, or right down on, full-fat dairy produce, replacing it with low-fat dairy produce and more pulses, nuts and seeds. For more tips on a healthy vegetarian diet, see below. You are now ready to start the six-week plan.

Here are some more tips to help prevent your digestive system from complaining:

- Chew all food thoroughly.
- Eat slowly.
- Make sure pulses are thoroughly cooked before eating. Some pulses, particularly red kidney beans, are toxic if not boiled for at least 10 minutes before using in your recipe. Canned beans are fine.
- Vegetables, fruits and pulses can be puréed to make them more easily digestible.
- Don't peel vegetables and fruit unless absolutely necessary. Buy organic, wash well and scrub if necessary.

Adding variety and taste

So you've cut out meat and cut down on dairy products – but if you're doing the thing properly, you will be eating **MORE** fruits, vegetables, pulses, whole grains, nuts, seeds and so on. So in fact you are adding more foods to the diet than you are taking away. There are dozens of different varieties of pulses alone, each with its own interesting texture and flavour.

All these plant foods are delicious, especially if you buy good quality, fresh food, preferably organic, and if you cook them with a bit of imagination. Fresh or dried herbs and spices, tomato sauces and so on all add flavour and versatility to your meals. The recipes and meal suggestions in the plan will help you to enjoy your diet.

It is worth considering buying organic fruits and vegetables as they will form a large part of your diet. They are guaranteed free from additives, hormones, pesticides, etc. and will help your overall health, long term. I think they also taste better.

For more information on vegetarian eating, diet planning, shopping, vegetarian nutrition in the young, pregnant and elderly, contact the Vegetarian Society (telephone 0161 928 0793).

Coping with a lone 'veggie' in the family

Whether that 'veggie' is you, or another family member, at first it seems like a lot of bother to cook two sets of meals. In fact it needn't present much extra work at all. During the day, most families eat separately anyway, so really it is just the evening meal that concerns us.

For a healthy family you would be well advised to encourage meat-eaters to eat more vegetables and pulses, in any event. Most meat-eaters will welcome one or two vegetarian meals a week – things like pizzas, pasta dishes, curries and so on are ideal as the missing meat is hardly noticed.

If you're eating fish, that's another two or three meals a week catered for. On the remaining three or so nights you can cook a basic vegetarian meal (a casserole or pie, for instance) and add chicken, lamb fillet, pork tenderloin or so on, to the meat-eater's portion.

Another tip for lone vegetarians is to cook a two-serving portion (as most of the recipes in this book are) then freeze the remaining portion for another night. This saves you time, too.

A few nutrition notes

Meat replacers When you give up meat you need to replace the nutrients it provided in your diet. The main ones of importance are protein, iron and B vitamins.

PROTEIN is present in a wide variety of vegetarian and demi-vegetarian foods including low-fat dairy, pulses, fish, eggs, protein replacers such as Quorn (made from a mushroom-like substance) and tofu (made from soya beancurd). Many other foods also contain reasonable amounts of protein, such as potatoes and other vegetables, grains, bread, nuts and seeds. A varied diet will ensure adequate protein. In fact, many meat-eaters get far more protein than they need and this can actually have drawbacks.

IRON is found in the vegetarian diet in dark leafy greens, some dried fruits, whole grains, pulses, spices, egg yolk and many other foods. Again, a varied diet including plenty of natural wholefoods will ensure a plentiful supply of iron. Another good idea is to eat a vitamin C-rich food (or drink) with each meal to help iron absorption – say, an orange juice with a boiled egg. Some iron-rich foods handily come ready with their own vitamin C – such as dark leafy greens! Also avoid tea and coffee with a meal as they can hinder absorption.

B VITAMINS are a group of six vitamins that work together in the body. They are found in varying quantities in a wide variety of foods including whole grains, pulses, nuts, seeds, eggs, vegetables, mushrooms, Marmite and dairy produce. Again, variety and regular meals are the key to adequate B intake.

DAIRY REPLACERS A good vegetarian diet, as we've seen, is one that doesn't rely too heavily on dairy produce, especially full-fat dairy produce. However, in cutting back on dairy items, you need to be sure to find other good sources of calcium in the diet. Low-fat dairy produce contains as much calcium as high-fat dairy produce, so unless going vegan, don't give up low-fat dairy altogether – regular daily skimmed milk and low-fat yogurt is a very good idea, and I would say almost vital for all women and teenagers (to help build and keep bone mass and help to prevent osteoporosis). If you don't eat dairy produce, choose calcium-fortified soya milk and yogurt (some brands aren't fortified with calcium).

Other good sources of calcium are seaweed, tofu, pulses, nuts, leafy greens, dried figs, apricots, muesli and broad beans. White bread is fortified with calcium and so contains more than wholemeal bread – but white bread misses out on the high fibre and vitamin content of wholemeal bread so perhaps a compromise – some white, some wholemeal – may be the answer. Lesser amounts of calcium are found in a variety of other plant foods, so again, it is important to have a varied diet with plentiful supplies of fresh vegetables. If you eat fish, sardines and whitebait are a good source of calcium in the bones.

And lastly ... If you are vegetarian, or going vegetarian, for your health, it may not worry you to eat some items containing animal by-products, e.g. some low-fat yogurts contain gelatine (a by-product of cattle) and many cheeses contain rennet (ditto). All kinds of foods may contain small amounts of non-vegetarian additives, from stock cubes to margarines.

But if it does worry you, you need to read labels avidly and perhaps ask your usual supermarket for a list of their products which are vegetarian.

What to do

Read this page before you begin the diet.

Every day pick a Breakfast, a Lunch, an Evening Meal and a Snack or Drink from the choices. When bread or toast is mentioned, unless otherwise specified it is a slice of wholemeal bread from a large medium-cut loaf spread with a little low-fat spread.

In addition to the meals and snacks mentioned on the week to a page diet you also have:

Milk Allowance

Every day you have an allowance of 250ml skimmed milk or calcium-enriched soya milk. If you don't drink milk, have 150ml natural low-fat bio yogurt or calcium-enriched soya yogurt instead. Milk for breakfast cereals is on top of this allowance.

Unlimiteds

Every day you can add anything you like from the following list to your diet:

- *Drinks* Water, mineral water, herbal teas, weak tea and coffee, green tea.
- *Foods* Leafy green vegetables, fresh salad items including lettuce and other salad leaves, cucumber, onions, fresh herbs.
- *Condiments* Fresh or dried herbs and spices, lemon juice, lime juice, vegetarian Worcester sauce, light soy sauce, tomato purée, passata, vinegar, oil-free dressings.

Week's Treats

Same as page 49.

WEEK ONE

Notes

- Read the instructions on page 99 before beginning.
- You can swap the suggested fruits in the meals for other similar fruits if preferred – swapping citrus for another citrus, berries for another berry, and so on.
- Men should increase portion sizes of bread, potatoes, pasta, rice and cereals and have extra skimmed or soya milk.

Breakfasts

- 2 Weetabix, 125ml skimmed milk; 1 orange.
- 1 slice toast with low-sugar jam or marmalade; 25g (medium bowlful) All-Bran with 100ml skimmed milk; ½ pink grapefruit.
- 1 Müller Light fruit yogurt; 1 large banana.

Lunches

- Sandwich – 2 slices bread filled with half a 115g pack St Michael Mediterranean Pâté and unlimited salad; 1 large banana.
- Soup – 1 portion Curried Lentil and Vegetable Soup (see recipe page 107); 1 mini wholemeal pitta bread; 1 apple.
- Salad – 40g feta cheese with unlimited salad items; 1 medium wholemeal roll with low-fat spread; 1 Shape fruit yogurt; 1 slice melon.
- Takeout – 1 Weight Watchers Vegetable and Pasta Medley; 1 small banana.

Evening Meals

- Recipe – 1 portion Chilli Beans and Pasta (see recipe page 108); 1 orange.
- Quick recipe – 1 portion Eggs Florentine with Toast (see recipe page 109); 1 kiwi fruit.
- Easy – 60g (dry weight) wholewheat pasta of choice, cooked and topped with ⅓ (107g) jar Dolmio Pasta Sauce with Extra Mushrooms and 1 tablespoon grated half-fat mozzarella cheese; side salad; 1 apple.
- Fish – 1 portion frozen Cod in Parsley Sauce; 175g instant mashed potato or home-made mash using skimmed milk; 4 tablespoons peas; 1 medium portion broccoli.

Snacks

- Good handful sunflower seeds (15g).
- Good handful shelled nuts of choice (15g).
- Drink – 100ml natural low-fat bio yogurt blended with 75ml orange juice and 1 teaspoon runny honey.

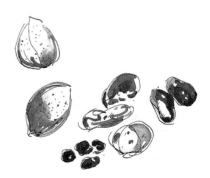

WEEK TWO

Notes

- Don't forget to include plenty of your 'unlimited' vegetables and salad items in your meals and snacks.
- You can choose meals from other weeks instead of those listed if you like, but choose from the same category – e.g., swap a Lunch with another Lunch, not with an Evening Meal.

Breakfasts

- 1 × 125ml tub low-fat natural bio yogurt topped with 25g muesli and 1 medium portion berry fruits or chopped nectarine and ½ medium banana plus 1 dessertspoon sesame seeds.
- 1 slice toast with 2 teaspoons honey; 1 large banana.
- 40g (large portion) All-Bran with 125ml skimmed milk; 1 apple.

Lunches

- Sandwich – 1 large wholemeal bap with low-fat spread, filled with half a pack St Michael Mushroom Pâté and unlimited salad; 1 Shape fromage frais.
- Soup – 1 whole pack New Covent Garden Tuscan Bean soup; 1 small wholemeal roll.
- Salad – 1 portion Noodle and Sesame Seed Salad (see recipe page 107); 1 orange.
- Takeout – 1 Boots Shapers Roast Vegetable and Ricotta Sandwich; 1 Boots Shapers Fresh Fruit Salad.

Evening Meals

- Recipe – 1 portion Aubergines with Couscous and Tomato Stuffing (see recipe page 112); 1 pear.
- Quick recipe – 1 portion Vegetarian Burgers (see recipe page 109); 40g (dry weight) brown rice, cooked; salad; 1 medium portion tzatziki made with low-fat natural bio yogurt mixed with chopped cucumber and seasoning to taste.
- Easy – 1 × 275g baked potato topped with 205g (half a large can) baked beans in tomato sauce; side salad; 1 orange.
- Takeout – 1 St Michael 95 per cent Fat Free Stonebake Vegetable Pizza; salad; orange.
- Fish – 1 portion Tuna Kedgeree (see recipe page 158); 1 apple.

Snacks

- 1 Sunblest Cracked Wheat Cr013 Crisproll with quarter pack (28g) St Michael Mediterranean pâté.
- 1 good handful (15g) sunflower seeds.
- Drink – 125ml skimmed milk blended with 120g strawberries and 1 teaspoon honey.

WEEK **THREE**

Notes

- Try to eat a wide range of different leafy vegetables and cook them lightly, or eat raw if possible, to retain maximum nutrients.

Breakfasts

- 40g (medium bowlful) Shreddies with 125ml skimmed milk; I orange.
- Medium bowl porridge made with half water and half skimmed milk; little extra skimmed milk to top; I teaspoon runny honey; I small banana or nectarine.
- I slice toast with low-sugar jam or marmalade; I Shape fruit yogurt; 125ml orange juice or I orange.

Lunches

- Sandwich – I wholemeal pitta bread filled with unlimited firm chopped salad items of choice plus 30g crumbled feta cheese, 4 stoned black olives and I dessertspoon olive oil plus lemon juice and seasoning to taste.
- Recipe – I portion Mozzarella and Courgette Toasties (see recipe page 112).
- Salad – I portion Cannellini Bean Pâté (see recipe page 106) with 3 dark rye Ryvitas and salad; I can Weight Watchers Country Vegetable soup; I kiwi fruit or plum.
- Takeout – Any egg and salad sandwich of 300 calories or less (read the label); I apple.

Evening Meals

- Recipe – I portion Spanish Chickpeas (see recipe page 110); 30g brown rice (dry weight), cooked; salad.
- Recipe – I portion Flat Mushrooms Stuffed with Pine Nut Risotto (see recipe page 108); 125ml tub low-fat bio yogurt with I teaspoon honey.
- Quick recipe – I portion Pasta and Grilled Halloumi Salad (see recipe page 106); I medium banana.
- Easy – I RealEat Vege Quarterpounder; 175g new potatoes or I wholemeal bap; I medium portion broccoli; 4 tablespoons peas, sweetcorn or broad beans; I teaspoon burger relish or 4 tablespoons home-made tomato sauce (see recipe page 107).
- Fish – I portion Salmon with Pesto and Spaghetti (see recipe page 59); I apple.

Snacks

- I apple and 4 pieces ready-to-eat dried apricot.
- 2 dark rye Ryvitas with 25g half-fat soft cheese and a raw carrot.
- I good handful (15g) sunflower or pumpkin seeds.

WEEK FOUR

Notes

- If you are avoiding gelatine, which is an animal product added to some diet yogurts, you can choose a small tub of low-fat bio yogurt instead of the diet fruit yogurts when mentioned, and add a little fruit purée.

Breakfasts

- 30g (medium bowl) oatbran flakes; 125ml skimmed milk; ½ pink grapefruit; 1 teaspoon sugar.
- 125ml low-fat bio yogurt; small orange and 1 apple chopped in; 10g All-Bran; 1 teaspoon brown sugar.
- 1 Müller Light yogurt; 1 large banana.

Lunches

- Sandwich – 2 slices bread with Marmite and unlimited salad; 1 × 150g pot Total Light Greek Yogurt with 1 teaspoon runny honey.
- Soup – 1 whole carton New Covent Garden Lentil and Tomato soup; 2 slices Melba toast.
- Salad – 4 dark rye Ryvitas with 1 × 115g pack St Michael Carrot and Coriander pâté; large salad; 1 kiwi fruit.
- Takeout – 1 Boots Shapers Spicy Bean Salad; 1 Boots Shapers Fruit Salad and 1 Boots Shapers strawberry yogurt.

Evening Meals

- Recipe – 1 portion Potato Gratin (see recipe page 110); salad; 1 satsuma.
- Quick Recipe – 1 portion Quorn and Sesame Stir-fry with Rice (see recipe page 110); 1 apple.
- Easy – 1 small baking tray filled with diced mixed vegetables – e.g. squash, courgette, red onion, sweet potato or red pepper, courgette, aubergine and onion, brushed with 1 tablespoon olive oil, seasoned and baked for 45 minutes or until tender, on 50g (dry weight) couscous, reconstituted and served with 1 tablespoon shaved pecorino.
- Takeout – 1 Quorn Chilli with Rice; 1 × 150g pot Ambrosia low-fat custard; 1 satsuma.
- Fish – 1 portion Swordfish and Red Pepper Kebabs (see recipe page 60); salad.

Snacks

- As Week 1.

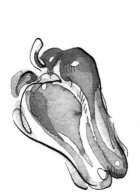
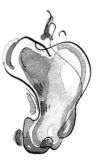

WEEK **FIVE**

Notes

- Don't forget to plan your week's menus in advance and stock up on plenty of healthy snacks so that you aren't caught hungry!

Breakfasts

- 2 Weetabix; 125g berries; 125ml skimmed milk; 1 heaped teaspoon sesame seeds.
- 1 slice toast with 1 medium egg, boiled or poached; 125ml orange juice or 1 orange.
- 1 × 150ml tub Total Light Greek Yogurt with 1 teaspoon runny honey; 1 medium banana.

Lunches

- Sandwich – 1 wholemeal pitta bread filled with 50g (2 level tablespoons) hummus (preferably home-made by puréeing canned chickpeas with lemon juice, olive oil, seasoning and a little light tahini paste, otherwise buy good quality hummus from a delicatessen) and unlimited firm chopped salad items of choice; 1 orange.
- Soup – 1 whole carton New Covent Garden Carrot and Coriander soup; 1 small wholemeal roll.
- Hot – ½ 410g can baked beans in tomato sauce on 40g slice wholemeal toast with low-fat spread; 1 medium banana.
- Hot – 1 portion Ratatouille (see recipe page 111) with 1 large egg, poached or griddled; 1 small wholemeal roll.

Evening Meals

- Recipe – 1 portion Aubergine and Lentil Curry (see recipe page 111); 1 ready-to-eat poppadom.
- Recipe – 1 portion Mushroom and Quorn Pie (see recipe page 113); 125g boiled potatoes; 1 medium portion carrots; plenty of leafy greens.
- Easy – 1 portion Macaroni and Broccoli Bake (see recipe page 108); 1 medium banana.
- Takeout – St Michael Cheese Ravioli in Tomato Sauce; salad; 1 slice bread.
- Fish – 1 medium trout (about 250g), grilled or otherwise cooked without added fat and sprinkled with 1 dessertspoon flaked toasted almonds; 175g new potatoes; 1 medium portion mangetout; 1 slice melon.

Snacks

- As Week 2.

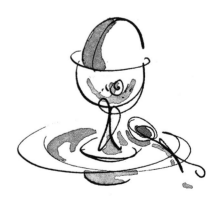

WEEK SIX

Notes

- After the end of this week, turn to Chapter 10 for what to do next.

Breakfasts

- 1 medium bowl porridge made with water with 4 ready-to-eat chopped apricots stirred in and 100ml skimmed milk to cover; 1 teaspoon runny honey.
- 1 medium bowlful Just Right with 125ml skimmed milk and 4 ready-to-eat dried stoned prunes chopped in; ½ pink grapefruit.
- 1 Müller Crunch Corner bio yogurt Honey and Muesli variety; ½ pink grapefruit.

Lunches

- Hot – 1 × 250g baked potato topped with 1 medium hard-boiled egg, chopped and stirred into 2 tablespoons whole-milk yogurt, topped with cress; side salad; 1 kiwi fruit or satsuma.
- Soup – 1 whole can Baxter's Carrot, Onion and Chickpea soup; 60g slice French bread with low-fat spread; 1 plum or 100g berries.
- Salad – Half a 170g pot fresh chilled guacamole with a selection of crudités and 1½ slices toast cut into fingers; 1 Shape fruit fromage frais.
- Takeout – 1 Findus French Bread Pizza, cheese and tomato variety; salad.

Evening Meals

- Recipe – 1 portion Cobbler Topped Goulash (see recipe page 113); 1 Shape fruit fromage frais.
- Quick Recipe – 1 portion Quick Pasta Gratin (see recipe page 106); salad; 1 medium banana.
- Quick Recipe – 1 portion Stir-fried Peppers and Egg (see recipe page 67); 1 Shape fruit fromage frais.
- Easy – 2-egg omelette cooked in a non-stick pan with a little low-fat spread, filled with chopped mushrooms; 100g oven chips or 1 pack microchips; 4 tablespoons peas or salad.
- Takeout – 1 Quorn Balti Jalfrezi with Naan Bread; 1 apple.
- Fish – 100g salmon fillet or steak marinated in 1 tablespoon Lea and Perrins 5-Minute Marinade Thai Coriander, Coconut and Lime, then grilled; 175g new potatoes or 4 tablespoons cooked long-grain rice; medium portion broccoli; 75g Weight Watchers Raspberry Swirl Iced Dessert or 1 French-style set yogurt.

Snacks

- As Week 3.

TOP 20 SLIMMERS' MEAT-FREE RECIPES

CANNELLINI BEAN PÂTÉ

Serves 4
113 calories and 5.5g fat per portion

1 can cooked cannellini beans, drained

1 clove garlic, crushed

1 tablespoon light tahini paste

Juice of ½ lemon

1 level teaspoon ground cumin

1 tablespoon olive oil

Salt and pepper

Blend all ingredients together in an electric blender or pound with pestle and mortar. Chill before serving.

PASTA AND GRILLED HALLOUMI SALAD

Serves 2
386 calories and 19g fat per portion

100g (dry weight) pasta shapes

1½ tablespoons olive oil

1 lemon

Salt and pepper

1 tablespoon chopped basil

75g Halloumi cheese, cut into four slices

2 medium tomatoes

8 black stoned olives, halved

1 small red onion, chopped

4cm piece cucumber, chopped

Boil the pasta in salted water until cooked; drain.

Meanwhile, combine the oil with the juice from a quarter of the lemon, the basil and the salt and pepper (use only a little salt as the cheese is quite salty). Heat the grill and, when the pasta is nearly ready, grill the cheese slices until flecked with brown, turn and grill the other side. While the cheese is grilling, drain the pasta and combine with the other salad ingredients and the dressing. Finally crumble the grilled Halloumi into the salad and serve immediately with lemon wedges.

QUICK PASTA GRATIN

Serves 2
360 calories and 13g fat per portion

80g (dry weight) short spaghetti

4 large tomatoes (about 400g in all)

1 dessertspoon olive oil

100g mushrooms, sliced

1 clove garlic, crushed

Salt and pepper

½ pack Napolina Creamy Lasagne Bake Sauce

2 tablespoons breadcrumbs

2 tablespoons grated Parmesan cheese

1 tablespoon finely chopped basil

Boil the spaghetti in salted water until cooked, drain.

Meanwhile, cut the tomatoes into 8 pieces each and sauté them in the oil in a non-stick frying pan with the mushrooms and garlic for a few minutes to soften. Season to taste. Tip the spaghetti into a two-serving size gratin dish (or individual gratin dishes) and cover with the tomato mixture, then pour over the creamy sauce. Mix the breadcrumbs, cheese and basil together in a bowl, then sprinkle evenly over the top. Grill under a medium high heat for a few minutes until browned.

NOODLE AND SESAME SEED SALAD

Serves 2
298 calories and 16g fat per portion

75g (dry weight) fine egg thread noodles

50g mangetout

75g fresh beansprouts

4 spring onions, halved lengthways

I medium red pepper, deseeded and finely sliced

50g Chinese leaves or Cos lettuce, thinly sliced

100g mushrooms, sliced

I tablespoon light soy sauce

I dessertspoon lime juice

I dessertspoon sesame seed oil

I dessertspoon toasted sesame seeds

Soak the noodles in boiling water for 3–4 minutes or as instructed on the packet, then drain.

Meanwhile, blanch the mangetout for I minute, drain and refresh with cold water. In a bowl, mix together all the vegetables. Mix the soy sauce, lime juice, sesame seed oil and sesame seeds and toss with the vegetables. Serve the vegetables lightly mixed into the noodles.

CURRIED LENTIL AND VEGETABLE SOUP

Serves 2
215 calories and 8.5g fat per portion

I tablespoon corn or groundnut oil

I medium onion, chopped

I level dessertspoon mild curry powder

450ml vegetable stock

I dessertspoon tomato purée

50g (dry weight) green lentils

100g cauliflower florets

2 medium carrots, chopped

I stick celery, chopped

Few sprigs parsley

Salt and black pepper

Heat the oil in a non-stick saucepan and add the onion and curry powder. Stir-fry for a few minutes. Add the rest of the ingredients, bring to a simmer, and cook gently for 40 minutes or until the lentils and all the vegetables are tender. You can serve the soup like this, or for a thicker soup you can remove half of it to an electric blender, blend, then return the blended soup to the pan, stirring in well and reheating.

TOMATO SAUCE

Serves 4
60 calories and 3.5g fat per portion

I tablespoon olive oil

I medium onion, finely chopped

I large clove garlic, crushed

I × 400g can chopped tomatoes

I level tablespoon tomato purée

I teaspoon brown sugar

I dessertspoon lemon juice

A little tomato juice or passata

Salt and black pepper

Heat the oil in a non-stick saucepan and stir the onion in it until softened. Add the garlic and stir again for a few minutes. Add chopped tomatoes with their juice, tomato purée, sugar and lemon juice, stir well and simmer for 30 minutes, stirring from time to time. You can add some tomato juice or passata or even water if the sauce gets too thick. When you have a rich sauce, season to taste. You can add spices or herbs as needed, depending upon the recipe the sauce is required for, or what it is to accompany.

MACARONI AND BROCCOLI BAKE

Serves 2
348 calories and 10.5g fat per portion

80g (dry weight) macaroni

110g broccoli

1 medium red pepper, deseeded and cut into thin strips

50g petit pois

200g 8 per cent fat fromage frais

100ml skimmed milk

Salt and pepper

25g half-fat grated mozzarella cheese

Boil the macaroni in salted water until cooked; drain.

Meanwhile, cut the broccoli into small florets and boil them with the red pepper in a little water. Add the peas towards the end of cooking time. When all are tender; drain. Beat together the fromage frais with the milk until you have a smooth sauce the consistency of custard, adding salt and pepper to taste (add a little more skimmed milk if necessary).

Toss the macaroni with the fromage frais mixture and the vegetables and tip into a shallow two-serving baking dish. Sprinkle the cheese on top and bake at 180°C/375°F/Gas 5 until golden and bubbling.

CHILLI BEANS AND PASTA

Serves 2
398 calories and 9g fat per portion

80g (dry weight) pasta bows

1 dessertspoon olive oil

1 medium onion, finely chopped

1 clove garlic, crushed

1 × 400g can cooked mixed beans in spicy pepper sauce
  (see note)

100ml passata

200g mixed peppers in tomato dressing (see note)

25ml stock

1 teaspoon chopped oregano

50g half-fat mozzarella cheese, thinly sliced

2 tablespoons breadcrumbs

Boil the pasta in salted water until cooked; drain.

Meanwhile, heat the oil in a non-stick pan and sauté the onion and garlic until softened. Now mix the onions with the beans, passata, peppers, stock, oregano and toss with the drained pasta. Tip into a two-serving gratin dish or individual gratin dishes and top with the mozzarella and breadcrumbs. Grill or bake until the top is golden and bubbling.

NOTE *If you can't find these beans, use a can of plain mixed beans, drained, and use extra passata (about 100ml) mixed with some ground chilli to taste.*

NOTE *If you can't find these peppers, use peppers canned in water or brine, drained, and add 1 level dessertspoon tomato purée to the recipe instead.*

FLAT MUSHROOMS STUFFED WITH PINE NUT RISOTTO

Serves 2
362 calories and 16g per portion

1 dessertspoon olive oil

4 spring onions, chopped

1 small clove garlic, chopped

90g (dry weight) risotto rice

20g pine nuts

200g chopped canned tomatoes

225ml vegetable stock

Salt and pepper

Chopped basil or flat-leafed parsley

4 large flat mushrooms

2 tablespoons grated Parmesan cheese

Heat the oil in a non-stick frying pan and add the onions, garlic and rice, stir well for a minute or two, then add the pine nuts, tomatoes and stock to the pan. Stir again, bring to simmer and cook gently for 20 minutes or until the rice is tender and most of the liquid absorbed. Season to taste and stir in the basil. Destalk the mushrooms and fill the mushrooms' cavities with the risotto. Sprinkle the cheese over and place the mushrooms in a shallow baking dish just big enough to take them. Bake at 200°C/400°F/Gas 6 for 20 minutes or until the mushrooms are tender, covering with foil if the rice looks like drying out.

EGGS FLORENTINE WITH TOAST

Serves 2
401 calories and 19g fat per portion

400g washed spinach

2 large free-range eggs

2 teaspoons French mustard

Salt and pepper

½ pack Napolita Creamy Lasagne Bake Sauce

50g grated half-fat mozzarella cheese

1 tablespoon grated Parmesan cheese

2 medium slices wholemeal bread

A little low-fat spread

Cook the spinach in a very little water until wilted. Chop if necessary and divide between two gratin dishes, spreading over the bases completely and making a well in the centre of each. Break an egg into each well. Beat the mustard and seasoning into the sauce and pour half over each dish, covering the egg and spinach completely. Top with the mozzarella and Parmesan and bake for 15 minutes at 200°C/400°F/Gas 6 by which time the egg white should be just set and the yolk still runny.

Toast the bread, spread with the low-fat spread and serve the eggs Florentine with the toast.

VEGETARIAN BURGERS

Serves 2
268 calories and 8.5g fat per portion

1 x 400g can chickpeas, drained

1 medium onion, finely chopped

1 whole canned sweet red pepper, well drained

1 clove garlic, chopped

½ teaspoon each ground cumin and coriander seed

1 pinch chilli powder

1 level dessertspoon finely chopped coriander leaf

Salt and pepper

1 egg white, beaten

1 dessertspoon corn oil

A little flour for coating

Mash the chickpeas in a bowl, or blend for a few seconds in an electric blender, without overblending as you still want some texture to the peas. In a bowl, combine the chickpea purée with the onion, pepper, garlic, spices, coriander leaf, seasoning and egg white. Using your hands, form into four patties, firming well. Heat the oil in a non-stick frying pan, coat the burgers in a little flour, and fry over a medium heat for 4–5 minutes each side or until the patties are golden. Serve immediately.

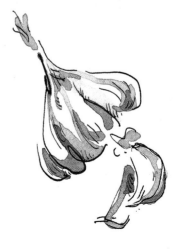

SPANISH CHICKPEAS

Serves 2
290 calories and 10g fat per portion

1 tablespoon olive oil

1 medium onion, chopped

1 clove garlic, crushed

1 small green pepper, deseeded and chopped

1 fresh green chilli, deseeded and chopped

1 level teaspoon each ground cumin and oregano

200g chopped canned tomatoes

200g (drained weight) canned chickpeas

75g (drained weight) canned red kidney beans

75g frozen sweetcorn

Salt and pepper

Heat the oil in a non-stick lidded frying pan and sauté the onion until soft and just turning golden. Add the garlic and pepper and stir a while longer, then add the chilli, cumin and oregano, and stir for a minute. Add the tomatoes, chickpeas, kidney beans and sweetcorn, stir well, bring to a simmer and cook, covered, for 20 minutes. Season to taste and serve.

POTATO GRATIN

Serves 2
397 calories and 12.5g fat per portion

425g old potatoes

1 tablespoon olive oil

1 medium red onion, thinly sliced

1 tablespoon finely chopped parsley

Salt and pepper

25g (dry weight) light sosmix

200ml skimmed milk

50ml vegetable stock

75g 8 per cent fat fromage frais

Peel the potatoes and slice into 0.5 cm slices. Parboil in salted water for 5 minutes, then drain and arrange half the slices in a two-serving size baking dish. Heat the oil in a non-stick frying pan and fry the onions until just turning golden. Add the parsley, seasoning and sosmix and stir for a minute or two, then spoon some onion mixture over the potatoes. Repeat the layers, then pour over the milk mixed with the stock and finish with dabs of fromage frais dotted all over. Bake at 160°C/325°F/Gas 3 for 1½ hours or until everything is tender (use a skewer to test) and the top is golden. Should the bake seem too dry towards the end of cooking, a very little stock can be carefully poured over.

QUORN AND SESAME STIR-FRY WITH RICE

Serves 2
405 calories and 17.5g fat per portion

85g (dry weight) long-grain or fragrant rice

1 dessertspoon groundnut oil

225g Quorn pieces

200g mix of baby sweetcorn, carrots and fine beans or mangetout

1 dessertspoon sesame oil

2 Little Gem lettuces, each quartered

1 tablespoon sesame seeds

1 tablespoon soy sauce

1 knob fresh ginger, peeled and chopped

1 clove garlic, chopped

Salt and black pepper

Boil the rice according to pack instructions. Halfway through cooking time, heat the groundnut oil in a non-stick frying pan and fry the Quorn pieces until they are golden on all sides. Remove with a slotted spoon. Add the baby vegetables and sesame oil and stir-fry for a few minutes, then return the Quorn to the pan with the lettuce, sesame seeds, soy sauce, ginger and garlic, and stir for a few minutes more, adding a little water or vegetable stock if the stir-fry looks too dry. Season to taste and serve the stir-fry with the cooked rice.

RATATOUILLE

Serves 2
150 calories and 7g fat per portion

1 tablespoon olive oil

1 large onion, sliced

1 clove garlic, crushed

1 large red pepper, deseeded and sliced

2 small courgettes (about 100g), sliced

1 small aubergine, sliced

1 × 200g can peeled tomatoes, roughly chopped

1 level teaspoon ground coriander seed or oregano or basil leaf

Salt and pepper

Heat the oil in a medium flameproof casserole and sauté the onion for a few minutes to soften. Add the garlic, pepper, courgettes and aubergine, stir and allow to cook over a very low heat for 30 minutes or so, stirring from time to time. Add the tomatoes and coriander, cover and simmer gently for another 30 minutes. The ratatouille is cooked when the vegetables are tender and the dish is very moist. Season to taste before serving.

NOTE *Good as a side dish with an omelette or the Vegetarian Burgers (recipe page 109), or as a main course topped with poached egg or grated cheese. Also makes a vegan main course on a bed of bulghar wheat.*

AUBERGINE AND LENTIL CURRY

Serves 2
397 calories and 12.5g fat per portion

1 tablespoon groundnut oil

1 large onion, sliced

1 medium yellow pepper, deseeded and sliced

1 large aubergine, about 325g

1 tablespoon biryani curry paste

175g cooked brown lentils or 50g dry weight lentils

50g (dry weight) basmati rice

400ml vegetable stock

200g canned chopped tomatoes

1 dessertspoon tomato purée

A little lemon juice

Salt and pepper

2 tablespoons natural low-fat bio yogurt

Chopped coriander leaf, to serve

Heat the oil in a non-stick lidded frying pan and sauté the onion until soft and just turning golden. Add the pepper and stir for a few minutes. Cut the aubergine into bite-sized pieces and add to the pan with the curry paste; stir for a minute. Add the lentils, rice, stock, tomatoes and tomato purée and stir well. Bring to a simmer, cover and cook gently for 40 minutes or until the vegetables are tender and the rice is cooked, stirring once or twice during cooking time and adding a little more stock towards the end of cooking time if necessary.

To serve, add a dash of lemon juice and seasoning as necessary and drizzle the yogurt over.

MOZZARELLA AND COURGETTE TOASTIES

Serves 2
357 calories and 8.5g fat per portion

8 cherry tomatoes, halved

I small red onion, peeled and cut vertically into eight
  wedges

I large or 2 small courgettes, sliced diagonally

2 dessertspoons olive oil

Salt and black pepper

2 × 75g slices rustic Mediterranean-style olive bread
  (e.g. ciabatta)

50g half-fat mozzarella cheese, thinly sliced

Heat the grill and place the tomatoes, onion pieces
and courgette slices on the grill pan. Drizzle over
I dessertspoon of olive oil and season. Grill under a
high heat for a few minutes until turning brown. Brush
one side of each of the bread slices with the rest of
the olive oil and add the bread to the pan, oil side up,
until lightly toasted. Remove pan from heat and
arrange the vegetables and the cheese slices on the
toast slices so that the vegetables are partially
covered by the cheese. Return to the grill and heat
until the cheese is bubbling. Serve.

AUBERGINES WITH COUSCOUS AND TOMATO STUFFING

Serves 2
384 calories and 9g fat per portion

I very large aubergine (about 400g)

150ml vegetable stock

75g (dry weight) quick-cook couscous

I tablespoon olive oil

I medium onion, chopped

I medium green pepper, deseeded and chopped

I clove garlic, crushed

25g sultanas

200g canned whole tomatoes drained of juice, roughly
  chopped

I pinch sugar

I level teaspoon allspice

100g cooked chickpeas

Salt and black pepper

100ml passata diluted with a little water

Chopped fresh coriander, to garnish

Halve the aubergine and remove the flesh, leaving a
thick shell. Leave upside down on kitchen paper while
you make the stuffing. Boil the stock and soak the
couscous in it for a few minutes.

Meanwhile, heat the oil and sauté the onion until
soft. Add the pepper and garlic and sauté again for a
few more minutes. Chop the aubergine flesh, then
add it with the sultanas, tomatoes, sugar, allspice and
chickpeas to the pan, and cook for a few more
minutes, stirring well and adding a little vegetable
stock if the mixture gets too dry. Off the heat, stir in
the couscous and season to taste. Place the
aubergine shells in a just-big-enough baking pan, fill
with the couscous mixture and pour the diluted
passata into the bottom of the pan. Cover loosely
with kitchen foil and bake at 200°C/400°F/Gas 6 for
25 minutes or until the aubergine shells are tender
when pierced with a knife or skewer. Garnish with
chopped coriander to serve.

NOTE *If there is any leftover stuffing which won't fit into the
aubergine shells, keep it in a covered container in the
refrigerator for a day or two. It will make a nice cold salad
snack at lunchtime.*

COBBLER TOPPED GOULASH

Serves 2
399 calories and 12g fat per portion

1 dessertspoon corn or groundnut oil

1 large leek, thinly sliced

1 medium courgette, thinly sliced

1 clove garlic, crushed

1 level dessertspoon Hungarian paprika

50g sliced mushrooms

275g (drained weight) cooked mixed pulses

100ml vegetable stock

100ml passata

Salt and black pepper

80g wholemeal self-raising flour

1 teaspoon baking powder

1 level teaspoon mixed dried herbs

20g half-fat Anchor butter

2 tablespoons low-fat natural yogurt

In a medium flameproof casserole, heat the oil and stir-fry the leek, courgette and garlic for a few minutes to soften. Add the paprika and stir for a minute, then mix in the mushrooms, pulses, stock, passata and seasoning, stir well, bring to simmer, cover and cook for 30 minutes or so in a hot oven, 200°C/400°F/Gas 6.

Meanwhile, make a scone topping by mixing together the flour, baking powder, a little salt and herbs and rubbing in the butter. Stir in the yogurt and bind together; knead gently on a floured board. Shape into six flat scones, using a cutter if you like and place on top of the casserole. Leaving the lid off, cook in the oven for a further 25 minutes or until the scones are golden. Serve immediately.

MUSHROOM AND QUORN PIE

Serves 2
342 calories and 13g fat per portion

1 tablespoon corn or sunflower oil

175g Quorn pieces

1 large onion, chopped

1 clove garlic, chopped

150g chestnut mushrooms, halved or sliced if large

1 sachet Colman's Bourguignon Sauce mix

1 teaspoon mixed herbs

3 oblong sheets filo pastry

1 teaspoon olive oil

Heat the oil in a non-stick frying pan and sauté the Quorn pieces until golden. Remove with a slotted spoon, then sauté the onion and garlic. Add the mushrooms to the pan and stir, then remove from heat. Make up the sauce according to pack instructions and mix into the Quorn mixture with the herbs. Divide the mixture between two individual pie dishes. Cut the sheets of filo in half, making six pieces in all. Put two sheets on each pie, crunching them up slightly, then brush the remaining two sheets with the olive oil and arrange one on top of each pie. Bake at 190°C/375°F/Gas 5 for 15 minutes or until the topping is golden.

CASE HISTORY

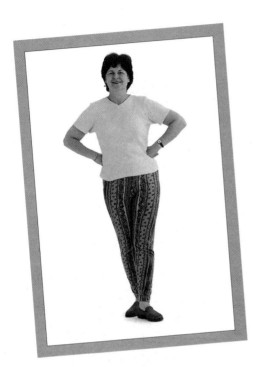

SUE REISS

AGE: **52**
STATUS: **Married; three teenage daughters**
OCCUPATION: **Freelance art gallery publicist**
HEIGHT: **5 ft 2 ins**
start weight: **10 st 6 lb**
WEIGHT AFTER SIX WEEKS: **9 st 10 lb**
START BMI: **27.7**
BMI AFTER SIX WEEKS: **25.8**
START STATISTICS: **37–32½–40½**
STATISTICS AFTER SIX WEEKS: **36½–30½–39**

Sue wrote to me saying that her whole life is one long rush – not only does she have three daughters and a part-time job as a publicist, she also sings with a jazz group and has other family commitments.

At only 5 ft 2 ins, Sue had managed to stay slim all her life without any problems, but once her menopause began, the weight gradually came on and Sue didn't know what to do about it. 'I recently tried a slimming club but it was too boring and I objected to paying to be weighed, but I thought that if I didn't do anything about my size and shape, it would be too late. I didn't want to end up like my mother – with a bad back, unable to walk far, and flabby.'

Sue disliked her tummy, her increasingly large bust, her upper arms – and wasn't pleased that she was hardly getting into a size 14 after being a size 10 not too many years ago.

Sue and I agreed that she wouldn't aim for a complete stone loss in six weeks, and that 10 lb or so would be a better goal. This is partly due to her lack of height (a ten-pound loss at 5ft 2ins is equivalent to a stone off someone a few inches taller), her age and her menopause. The wisdom is that menopause and HRT can cause weight gain, and although there is little hard evidence to support this, many women who have previously been slim do find it increasingly hard to maintain their previous weight around this time. As Chapters 1 and 2 explain, though, as women get older it is better not to aim for too low a weight, in any case.

Sue's BMI was a little high, though, at getting on for 28, and we knew that if she could lose 10 lb in the six weeks she would be almost down to the healthy 25 figure.

And a loss of 10 lb is exactly what she did achieve in the six weeks, by following the meat-free plan with the fish option. 'I hardly eat any red meat anyway, so I think I will like this plan,' Sue said at the start of the programme. 'Also, my husband has had heart problems and it will be good for him to eat more healthily, too.'

Eating a healthy breakfast, including fruit and milk or yogurt each morning – something Sue had not done previously – gave her a good start to the day and helped keep hunger at bay until lunchtime, when she would usually have salad or soup. Evening meals were varied and enjoyed by both Sue and husband Charles – 'We enjoyed your recipes – they were delicious.'

Sue had a week away in Portugal on holiday, where she stuck as far as possible to fish, salads and seafood, and swam and played tennis, and by the time she returned, found she had lost a little weight while away – and it continued to come off steadily through the six weeks.

'I wasn't expecting to lose much weight,' says Sue, 'so when I saw the weight coming off at a reasonable pace while I was still eating well, I was delighted and couldn't believe it.

'I probably didn't do as much exercise as I should have, but I did the mid-body tone up for my stomach regularly, swam, and walked using a walking machine. I shall carry on with the exercise as I feel much fitter and less sluggish now; I have more energy, I feel "bouncier" and my back is not as bad as it was.'

Sue is determined to keep up her new, healthier habits for life. Health **IS** Sue's main motivation – but the admiring comments she's received from the family since shedding a whole dress size have been no small bonus, either!

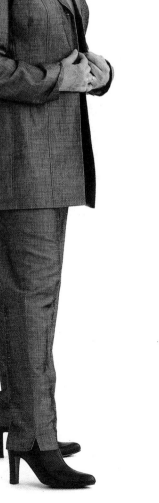

Debenhams' J. Taylor trousers, Debenhams' T-shirt and jacket, Littlewoods' boots

the business plan

'It isn't food that makes me fat,' said a colleague of mine recently. 'It's work!'

What he meant, of course, was that his working life involves so much eating and drinking that he feels it is his job, rather than any true gluttony on his part, that is keeping his girth at a steady 38ins.

And in truth, many careers these days entail what seems like an almost never-ending catalogue of lunches, dinners out, evenings entertaining at home, even power breakfasts. For others, life is spent travelling from one meeting to another and meals are grabbed in cafés, wine bars, from delis and on airlines and trains.

Because caterers and restaurant chefs don't, as a matter of course, feel obliged to provide healthy, calorie-controlled meals – after all, many lunch and dinner tables are booked by people for whom eating out is an occasional treat, and for whom a low-calorie meal would feel like poor value for money – I estimate that people who 'eat on the job' and feel they have little control over what is on their plates or in their mouths are probably eating in a typical 'business food' day at least 50 per cent more than they need to support a reasonable body weight. For men that could mean up to a total of 3,750 calories a day; for women up to 3,000.

Add to that the other two factors common among business people – too much alcohol and not enough exercise – and no wonder they find weight gain almost inevitable – and weight loss nearly impossible.

But I have to say that however often you have to eat out; however often you have to entertain; and however often you have to eat while travelling, a good deal of what you eat and drink is, in fact, down to *you* making the wrong choices. And that is the basis of this plan – showing you how to cut the calories without altering the way you operate.

For example, you wind up most lunchtimes in a roadside café with a fry-up at 1,000 calories. But there are much lower fat alternatives available for half those calories. What are they?

You discuss a contract over a quick meal in a pub. Which is going to do your waistline least harm – the curry and rice or the ham salad ploughman's?

You entertain a client in the evening and choose a Chinese restaurant. But for a lower-fat, lower-calorie meal, would the Italian place have been a better bet?

This plan arms you with the knowledge you need to make the right choices. It also aims to encourage you to realise that you can make those choices without starving and without seeming unsociable.

I also help you plan menus for home entertaining and provide several recipes which look and taste impressive but which can help you stick to a slimming programme.

And lastly there is a 'basic' plan to take advantage of those quieter days and days off to help the weight come off steadily over the weeks ahead.

Read on for more detail about how your six weeks on the Business Plan will work.

What to do

Every day all you do is decide whether you are going to be able to follow a **BASIC** day, a **BIG LUNCH OR BREAKFAST** day, or a **BIG EVENING** day.

BASIC days are for when you haven't any meals out planned and no entertaining at home. The **BASIC** day meal choices on pages 120–2 provide you with around 1,300 calories a day, and include items you can get from the take-away, sandwich shops and supermarket ready meals.

BIG LUNCH OR BREAKFAST days are just that – for when you have a working lunch or breakfast (or, indeed, a private occasion celebration), or when you are overnighting in a hotel and want to take full advantage of the 'free' full breakfast on offer. You can also use the big breakfast or lunch (up to 750 calories each) if you know you will be eating in a café or fast-food joint on the way to or from somewhere. You decide whether you are going to have a big lunch or a big breakfast (you can't have both on the same day!) and then choose from the comprehensive ideas on pages 123–5. On these days you are also allowed two further meals, and the days' menus provide you with approximately 1,500 calories altogether.

BIG EVENING days are for when you will be eating a full meal in a restaurant, or entertaining at home. These menus, on page 127, provide you with approximately 1,600 calories a day and allow for a three-course meal of up to 1,000 calories (or a two-course meal with wine), as well as two small meals during the rest of the day. You can, of course, choose to have your 1,000-calorie meal at lunchtime instead, and have one of the small meals in the evening that day.

As explained in the chapter introduction, I estimate that you may have been eating between 3,000 and 3,750 calories a day, and so the above plans will give you a very good calorie deficit which will certainly help you to shed weight steadily. The exact rate of loss will depend on you, your current weight and your schedule. But if you can manage, say, three **BASIC** days a week, two **BIG LUNCH** days and two **BIG EVENING** days that will give you an average daily calorie intake over a week of around 1,450.

Don't worry if any one week is different from this suggested plan – you may have a heavy week with five **BIG LUNCH** days and two **BIG EVENING** days and no **BASIC** days at all, for example. Even then, you should still lose some weight as long as you follow the guidelines for what to pick when you're eating out.

If you are now going to claim 'Well, that's no good, most days I have a big lunch *and* a big evening', I have to tell you that you need to examine, honestly, your lifestyle, your commitments, your work patterns, and your views on yourself, your needs and your future health.

Why do you have so many lunches and evening meals out? Are you absolutely sure these are all necessary to your business or your career? Could meetings be rescheduled for other times of day? Could you entertain informally in the office with sandwiches, takeout salads, etc.? Could you swap evening entertaining for breakfast meetings that will do less damage to your waistline? Treat your slimming programme like you do your work – with a bit more organisation and preplanning you probably can manage to cut down on at least 30 per cent of your meals out!

However, I do have one last trick up my sleeve for those of you who may find they do have the occasional day when they have to eat out twice. On such days, you simply follow a **BIG LUNCH** day. Choose a meal from the Big Lunch list for your largest meal of the day and then check down the 500-calorie meals list for your other meal out – you will find several items there that you will find on menus everywhere.

If that is impossible, as a last resort, choose two **BIG LUNCHES** on such days, which will add only an extra 250 calories to your day's intake, giving a day's total of 1,750 – still low enough to create a small calorie deficit.

And for people who often have lunch in cafés, etc. while travelling – please do consider taking your lunch with you; it will nearly always be a more reliable way of controlling your calorie and fat intake than relying on what you can find a hundred miles up the road.

More tips on all these subjects appear in the pages ahead.

EVERY DAY EXTRAS

Every day on the six-week plan, in addition to anything mentioned in the Basic, Big Lunch and Big Evening menus in the pages ahead, you can have:

Milk Allowance

A daily milk allowance of 125ml minimum for men and 200ml minimum for women. Milk for breakfast cereals is on top of this allowance.

The milk should be skimmed. This is for use in tea or coffee or as a drink on its own. If you don't want it, have one 125ml pot natural low-fat yogurt instead. This is especially important for women because of the calcium content.

Unlimiteds

- *Drinks* Water, mineral water, low-calorie mixers and fizzy drinks, tea or coffee with milk from allowance (no sugar), green tea, herbal teas, lemon juice.
- *Foods* Salad greens, cucumber, onions, any raw vegetables such as carrot, celery and any green leafy vegetables, cooked or raw.
- *Condiments* Fresh or dried herbs and spices, lemon juice, lime juice, Worcestershire sauce, light soy sauce, vinegar, oil-free French dressing, chilli sauce.

Fruit

When 'fruit' is mentioned within the plan, choose one portion of fruit of choice. If you choose a banana, make it a small one. A small fruit salad is fine, or a combination of fruits totalling what you'd consider to be an average portion is also fine – e.g. a plum and a kiwi fruit, or a plateful of mixed berries.

Bread

When 'one slice bread' is mentioned within the plan, unless otherwise stated, this means one slice of white or wholemeal bread from a large, medium-cut loaf with a little low-fat spread. This can of course be toasted if liked.

A Word About Alcohol

On this plan, half a bottle of wine or its equivalent is built into the **BIG EVENING** days – you can choose this instead of a starter or dessert. I haven't included a regular alcohol allowance in the **BIG LUNCH** days as I believe it is best to try to avoid drinking alcohol during the day – alcohol is a drug and a depressant and can impair decision making and performance and can also tend to make you indiscreet – all traits it is best to avoid if you are in business.

I have also not included alcohol in the **BASIC** days as it is on these days that we are paring unnecessary calories so that you lose weight steadily. However, the occasional glass of wine does feature in some of the evening meal suggestions on both the Big Lunch and the Basic plans, and an extra glass now and then won't do you any harm.

Tips about reducing your alcohol consumption appear on pages 129–30.

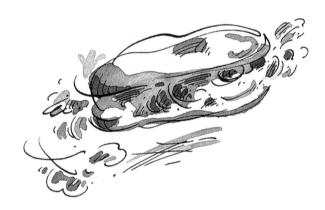

BASIC DAYS

- Follow this as often as possible during the next six weeks.
- Don't forget your milk allowance and 'unlimiteds' (see page 118).

Every day on the **BASIC**, pick a Breakfast, a Lunch, an Evening Meal and a Snack.

Breakfasts

- 40g (1 medium to large bowlful) any unsweetened breakfast cereal of choice, such as branflakes, cornflakes, Fruit'n Fibre, Special K or Start, with 125ml skimmed milk; 1 slice bread with low-sugar jam or marmalade.
- 1 x 125ml pot Danone Bio fruit flavoured yogurt with 25g muesli sprinkled in; 1 medium banana.
- 125ml low-fat natural bio yogurt topped with 1 level dessertspoon sesame seeds, 1 teaspoon runny honey, 1 portion fruit, chopped as necessary; 1 small slice bread with low-fat spread and low-sugar jam or marmalade or Marmite.
- 1 slice bread; ½ 200g pot Total Greek Yogurt; 1 portion fruit; 125ml orange juice.
- 50g muesli with 125ml skimmed milk; 1 portion fruit.
- 2 Weetabix with 125ml skimmed milk; 1 portion fruit; 1 level dessertspoon sunflower or sesame seeds.
- 1 medium egg, boiled or poached; 1 slice bread; 1 kiwi fruit or plum or satsuma; 25g All-Bran or Bran Buds with 75ml skimmed milk.
- 200g baked beans in tomato sauce on 1 slice toast; 125ml orange juice.
- 2 slices bread with low-sugar jam or marmalade or Marmite; 1 Shape diet fruit yogurt; 1 portion fruit.
- 1 Müller Crunch Corner yogurt; 1 large banana.

Snacks

- 1 Shape fruit yogurt; 1 dark rye Ryvita with Marmite.
- 1 large banana.
- 1 good handful sunflower seeds.
- 4 pieces ready-to-eat dried apricot or prune; 1 apple.
- 2 dark rye Ryvitas with 50g cottage cheese.
- 1 x 125ml tub low-fat natural bio yogurt with 1 teaspoon runny honey.
- 1 round crumpet with a little low-fat spread and low-sugar jam.
- 1 portion fruit; 1 small digestive biscuit.

Lunches Sandwiches

- 2 slices bread filled with 1 individual portion Bel Paese cream cheese or 2 slices extra-lean ham; 2 teaspoons sweet pickle; lettuce; 1 Shape fruit fromage frais; 1 portion fruit.
- 1 white pitta filled with 1 x 100g can tuna in brine or water, drained and mixed with chopped salad vegetables and 1 tablespoon Kraft Free Choice mayonnaise; 1 Shape fruit yogurt.
- 1 large wholemeal bap with low-fat spread filled with 2 slices lean turkey from vacuum pack, unlimited salad and 2 teaspoons cranberry sauce; 1 Prewett's Banana Bar.
- 2 slices bread filled with 40g half-fat Cheddar, tomato, cucumber; 1 Boots Shapers yogurt mousse, any flavour.
- 2 slices bread filled with 1 medium hard-boiled egg, unlimited salad, 1 dessertspoon Free Choice mayonnaise; 1 large banana.

Lunches Soups

- I whole carton New Covent Garden Tomato or Tomato and Lentil soup; I slice bread.
- I portion Curried Lentil and Vegetable Soup (see recipe page 107); I mini pitta; I portion fruit.
- I whole carton New Covent Garden Tuscan Bean soup; I small wholemeal roll with low-fat spread.
- I whole carton New Covent Garden Carrot and Coriander soup; I small wholemeal roll.
- I portion Watercress Soup (see recipe page 133); I wholemeal bap; I portion fruit.

Lunches Salads

- I medium cooked portion of chicken breast (skin removed) with unlimited salad items and either I small wholemeal roll or 125g cold new potatoes; I dessertspoon Free Choice mayonnaise or low-calorie vinaigrette; I plum or satsuma.
- 175g leftover cooked rice mixed with I handful (50g) cold chopped turkey or ham plus chopped raw salad vegetables, 25g chopped ready-to-eat dried apricots and oil-free French dressing to combine; I Shape fruit yogurt.
- 40g feta cheese, tomato, cucumber, pepper, onion and 4 black stoned olives; oil-free French dressing; I pitta; I portion fruit.
- I portion Noodle and Sesame Seed Salad (see recipe page 107); I portion fruit.
- 4 dark rye Ryvitas; I × 115g pot St Michael Carrot and Coriander Pâté; large salad; I portion fruit.

Lunches Hot

- 200g baked beans in tomato sauce on I slice toast; I tablespoon grated half-fat mozzarella cheese; I large banana.
- I large poached egg on I slice toast; I orange; I Quaker Harvest Chewy bar.
- I Findus French Bread Pizza, cheese and tomato flavour; I Shape fruit fromage frais; I portion fruit.
- I × 275g baked potato topped with 100g ready-made tzatziki; side salad; I portion fruit.
- I St Michael 95 per cent Fat-Free Stonebake Vegetable Pizza; salad.

Lunches Takeout

- Any one supermarket ready-made sandwich with 300 calories or less (check pack); I portion fruit.
- I McDonald's hamburger, regular (no cheese); I McDonald's pure orange juice.
- I take-away baked potato with baked bean filling; I portion fruit.
- St Michael Lite Layered Egg Salad; I St Michael Lite fruit yogurt; I portion fruit.
- I Boots Shapers triple sandwich pack; I fruit.

Evening Meals Recipe dishes

- I portion Moroccan Lamb with Couscous (see recipe page 65); I medium glass wine.
- I portion Pasta with Sardines and Sultanas (see recipe page 59); salad.
- I portion Salmon with Pesto and Spaghetti (see recipe page 59); salad; I portion fruit.
- I portion Chicken Curry (see recipe page 62) or Balti Curry (see recipe page 64); I medium glass wine.
- I portion Turkey with Egg Thread Noodles (see recipe page 63); I single measure spirits with calorie-free mixer.
- I portion Flat Mushrooms Stuffed with Pine Nut Risotto (see recipe page 108); I medium glass wine; I Shape fromage frais.

- 1 portion Aubergine and Lentil Curry (see recipe page 111); 1 average ready-made poppadom.
- 1 portion Mozzarella and Courgette Toasties (see recipe page 112); 1 banana.
- 1 portion Venison and Guinea Fowl Casserole (see recipe page 135); 4 tablespoons cooked bulghar wheat; broccoli and one other vegetable of choice.
- 1 portion Spiced Creamy Salmon with Lentils (see recipe page 133); 2 tablespoons cooked couscous.

Evening Meals Quick and Easy

- 175g beef steak, grilled, with 1 pack McCain Micro Chips; peas; 1 portion fruit.
- Birds Eye Cod Steak in crisp crunch crumb, grilled or baked; 225g mashed potato or 110g oven chips; peas or sweetcorn.
- 1 × 175g gammon steak, fat removed, grilled; 1 ring pineapple; 175g mashed potato or new potatoes; broad beans, peas or sweetcorn.
- 1 average chicken breast portion, brushed with ready-made basting sauce, baked or grilled; 5 tablespoons (cooked weight) rice or couscous; large side salad; 1 medium glass wine.
- 1 Quarterpounder Vegeburger, grilled or dry-fried; 1 large bap or 175g potatoes; sweetcorn; salad; 1 medium glass wine.
- 1 medium trout, cooked without fat, coated with 1 level tablespoon flaked toasted almonds; 200g new potatoes; 1 large portion mangetout; 1 portion fruit.
- 75g (dry weight) pasta of choice, cooked and topped with 1/3 jar (107g) Dolmio pasta sauce with extra mushrooms and 1 tablespoon grated Parmesan; side salad; 1 portion fruit.
- 2-egg omelette filled with 50g extra-lean diced ham; 100g pack McCain Micro Chips; large salad; 1 portion fruit.

- 2 taco shells warmed and filled with a mixture of 1 medium cooked chicken breast fillet (no skin), chopped and mixed with Old El Paso mild or hot taco sauce, sliced crisp lettuce, chopped tomato and onion, and topped with 1 good tablespoon ready-made guacamole and 1 tablespoon half-fat Greek yogurt; 1 medium glass wine.
- 110g (medium) salmon steak, grilled or dry-fried; with 150g new potatoes; peas; broccoli; 1 tablespoon Hollandaise sauce or mayonnaise; 1 medium glass wine.

Evening Meals Ready Meals

Add salad or leafy green vegetables to these if possible.

- Chilled counter – 1 St Michael Chicken Sag with Basmati Rice.
- Chilled counter – 1 St Michael Potato, Cauliflower and Broccoli Bake.
- Chilled counter – 1 St Michael Roast Beef, Yorkshire Pudding and Roast Potatoes.
- Frozen – 1 Sharwood's Thai Red Curry with Coconut Rice.
- Frozen – 1 Birds Eye MenuMaster Spaghetti Bolognese or Lasagne.

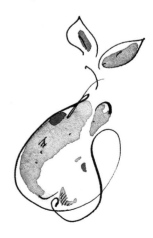

BIG LUNCH OR BREAKFAST DAYS

Decide whether you're going to have a Big Lunch or a Big Breakfast. Both contain up to 750 calories

Big breakfasts

Big breakfasts are suitable for all working breakfasts, hotel breakfasts, café breakfasts and Sunday brunches at home.

Big lunches

Big lunches are suitable for meals on the road, take-aways, cafés, wine bars, pubs, more casual restaurants such as steak bars and carveries and so on.

- With either choice, select also a 200-calorie Light Snack from the list below (at breakfast time if you're having a Big Lunch, or at lunchtime if you're having a Big Breakfast), and a 500-calorie Evening Meal.
- To give you more flexibility, you could of course have the 500-calorie meal at lunchtime and your Big Lunch in the evening, using your 200-calorie snack as breakfast. This would be useful if you are having a more casual meal out in the evening than those offered on the Big Evening plan.
- Don't forget your milk allowance and 'unlimiteds', too (see page 118).

200 CALORIE LIGHT SNACKS

Choose one a day

Breakfast snacks

- 1 individual box breakfast cereal with skimmed milk to cover; 1 small glass fresh fruit juice.
- 1 Shape Bio Twinpot yogurt, any variety; 1 large banana.
- 125g pot low-fat natural bio yogurt with small handful muesli stirred in; 4 pieces ready-to-eat dried apricot, chopped.
- 2 Weetabix with skimmed milk to cover; 1 plum or satsuma or kiwi fruit.
- 1 slice toast with low-sugar marmalade; 1 Shape fruit yogurt; 1 portion fruit.
- 125g pot low-fat natural bio yogurt with 1 teaspoon runny honey and 1 small banana chopped in.
- $\frac{1}{2}$ grapefruit; 1 large boiled egg; 1 slice bread.
- 1 Nutri-Grain morning bar; 1 Shape fruit yogurt or 1 portion fruit.
- 1 medium bowlful porridge made with skimmed milk and water; 1 teaspoon syrup or brown sugar; 1 portion fruit.
- Müller Fruit Corner yogurt; 1 small glass grapefruit juice.

Lunch snacks

- $\frac{1}{2}$ can wholewheat spaghetti in tomato sauce on 1 slice toast.
- 2 slices bread or toast with Marmite and salad.
- 5 tablespoons baked beans in tomato sauce on 1 slice toast.
- 2 dark rye Ryvitas with 2 triangles light cheese spread; 1 banana.

- I can Weight Watchers soup of choice; I small wholemeal roll.
- I Boots Shapers Tuna and Pasta Salad or Chinese-Style Chicken Salad.
- Any Boots Shapers sandwich 200 calories or less (check pack).
- I small chicken breast portion, cooked, skin removed; large salad with oil-free French dressing.
- I Lean Cuisine Snackpot (230g), Chicken and Prawn Creole or Chinese Noodle or Vegetable Balti variety.
- Sandwich of 2 slices bread from a small cut loaf with a little low-fat spread filled with salad and I small hard-boiled egg or 25g Edam or Brie.

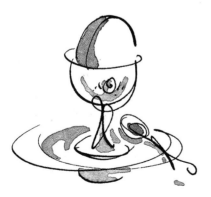

750-CALORIE BIG BREAKFASTS

Choose one of these or a Big Lunch, but not both.

NOTE 'Spread' is any margarine or butter, not low-fat. Medium bowl cereal is approx. 40g.

- I medium glass fresh juice; I medium bowlful any cereal (except muesli) with whole milk to cover; I fried egg; 2 rashers back bacon; grilled tomato; I slice toast and spread; marmalade or jam.
- I medium glass fresh juice or grapefruit segments in juice; I average (275g) grilled kipper; 2 slices toast with spread; marmalade or jam.
- I medium glass fresh fruit juice; I medium bowl cereal (except muesli) with fresh fruit salad or fruit compôte; whole milk to cover; 2 poached eggs on 2 slices toast with spread.
- I large sausage or I large slice black pudding; I fried egg; average portion baked beans; average portion fried mushrooms; 2 rashers back bacon; I slice fried bread.
- I medium bowlful (70g) muesli with whole milk to cover; 2 boiled eggs; 2 slices toast with spread; jam or marmalade.
- I medium bowlful natural yogurt with small portion cereal sprinkled over and medium portion fresh fruit salad or fruit compôte; scrambled eggs on I slice toast; 2 rashers back bacon or I rasher back bacon and extra slice toast.
- Selection of fresh fruits; 125ml tub fruit yogurt; 2 small croissants with spread and conserves.
- McDonald's Big Breakfast; McDonald's pure fruit juice.
- Little Chef Early Starter.
- Little Chef American Style Breakfast; fruit juice.

750-CALORIE BIG LUNCHES

Choose one of these or a Big Breakfast,
but not both.

- Café – Average cheese omelette; chips; peas.
- Café – 1 sausage; 2 fried eggs; chips.
- Steak house – 225g steak (don't eat fat); regular French fries; salad (no dressing); fresh fruit salad and cream or sorbet.
- Steak house – Harvester Chargrilled Salmon with fries; salad (no dressing).
- Burger bar – Burger King Cheeseburger Deluxe; regular French fries.
- Burger bar – McDonald's Big Mac; regular French fries.
- Little Chef – Vegetable Burger and Cheese or Quarterpounder Beefburger; chips; peas.
- Pizza bar – Pizza Express individual Pizza Margherita or Marinara or Mushroom.
- Mexican café – Chicken enchiladas; salad.
- Wine bar or pub – Cheese ploughman's.
- Wine bar or pub – Quiche; salad; chips.
- Wine bar or pub – Lasagne; small portion chips; salad (no dressing).
- Wine bar or pub – Baked potato with average serving of traditional ham and butter; salad.
- Wine bar or pub – Chilli con carne and rice; small roll or ½ pint beer or 1 glass wine.
- Wine bar or pub – Beef curry; rice; chutney.
- Take-away – Thai green chicken curry; rice.
- Take-away – Chinese – Chicken chow mein; 1 small spring roll.
- Take-away – Chinese – Chicken chop suey; plain soft noodles.
- Take-away – Chip shop – average portion cod in batter; regular chips.

500-CALORIE EVENING MEALS

Choose one of these a day.

At home hot meals

- Medium portion roast or grilled chicken (skin removed); fat-free gravy; 1 small baked potato; selection of vegetables, plainly cooked; 1 tablespoon stuffing or bread sauce.
- 4 slices lean roast beef; 1 individual Yorkshire pudding (frozen); ½ small baked potato; selection of vegetables, plainly cooked; fat-free gravy; 1 dessertspoon horseradish sauce.
- 3 slices leg of roast lamb or 2 trimmed lamb chops; medium portion (about 200g) new or boiled potatoes; selection of vegetables, plainly cooked; fat-free gravy; mint sauce.
- 1 whole carton New Covent Garden Lentil and Tomato or Broccoli and Stilton soup; 1 wholemeal bap; 1 portion fruit.
- 1 large individual skate, cod or other white fish portion, large, grilled, microwaved or baked; 200g new potatoes or 1 small baked potato; selection of vegetables plainly cooked, or salad; 1 portion fruit.

Home or away salads and sandwiches

- Medium portion lean ham or chicken (skin removed), 1 wholemeal roll with spread; large salad; 1 dessertspoon mayonnaise.
- Ploughman's – 75g slice French bread with spread; 40g Cheddar cheese; pickle; side salad without dressing; 1 apple.
- Pasta salad – average deli serving tuna, ham or chicken pasta salad; 1 portion fruit.

- 1 average take-away long baguette filled with salad and ham or chicken, or roast vegetables and feta cheese; 1 portion fruit (or you can make this at home).
- 1 average bap and spread, filled with 40g Brie and salad; 1 apple, 1 medium banana; 1 Shape fruit fromage frais.
- 1 Boots Shapers sandwich (or any other brand) 300 calories or less (check pack); 1 Müller Light fruit yogurt; 1 large banana.

Take-aways and restaurants

- 1 average doner kebab with salad.
- 1 average bacon sandwich.
- 1 McDonald's regular hamburger; regular French fries.
- 1 prawn chop suey; plain rice.
- 1 vegetable balti take-away; mini pitta bread.
- 1 chicken or prawn tandoori; plain rice.

Ready Meals

- 1 St Michael Cantonese Menu.
- 1 St Michael Low-fat Chicken and Rice Bowl; 1 apple.
- 1 Birds Eye Healthy Options Vegetable Indian Meal; 1 medium banana.

OR

You can also choose any meal from the *Evening Meals* list on the **BASIC** plan on page 120–2.

Tips to help you save calories

- If you see any visible fat on the food on your plate – e.g. on bacon, steak, etc. – leave it.
- If you are full before you have finished, leave the rest.
- If there is a choice of whole milk or skimmed, butter or low-fat spread, choose the lower-fat options.
- Ask for your salads undressed.
- Try to plan what you are going to have before you get to the café, wine bar, etc. That way you are less likely to be tempted by alternatives.

Avoid

You can eat almost anything if you allow for it within your day's calorie intake, as these pages prove. But here are some tips on what it may be best to avoid:

Breakfasts
- Fried mushrooms are very high in fat so unless you love them, leave them.
- Black pudding and fried sausages are also lethally high in calories, so if avoidable, stick with the grilled bacon. One slice of bread can soak up about 150 calories' worth of fat so save fried bread for a special treat.

Lunches
- Pies and pasties are some of the most fattening café items you can eat; so pick from the other items on the menu. Chips are always going to be quite high in calories, but the fatter the chip the less fat it will have absorbed, so if possible go for large chips rather than French fries or crinkle cuts.

Take-aways
- These should all be approached with caution. Many Chinese and Indian dishes can be swimming in fat. Burgers can be full of fat. Pizzas are mostly extremely high-calorie items. The take-aways given in the meal suggestions on these pages are some of the few that provide reasonable nutrition for not too many calories.

BIG EVENING DAYS

On these days, all you have to do is choose one 200-calorie Light Snack (see list pages 123–4); one Light Lunch (choose a lunch from the lunches list in the **BASIC** diet on pages 120–2) and then, if you are going out, a 1,000-calorie (approximately) three-course meal from the suggestions on these pages or, if entertaining at home, a three-course meal from the menus to cook at home (page 132). If you want half a bottle of wine, have it instead of either a starter or dessert (preferably dessert).

Of course, all restaurant recipes vary and these calorie counts can only be approximate. On pages 128–9 you will find more ideas on the best and worst dishes to pick in a variety of ethnic restaurants.

Three-course menus for dining out

Each of these contains approx. 1,000 calories.

INDIAN
Chicken tikka (starter portion)
Vegetable biryani
Fresh mango fruit salad

THAI
Hot and sour soup
Green chicken curry
Fried bananas (no batter)

CHINESE
Sweetcorn and crab soup
Chicken chop suey; steamed prawns with chilli and ginger
Small portion fried rice
Fresh lychees

ITALIAN
Melon or figs and Parma ham
Chicken cacciatore; salad
Ice cream selection

Mozzarella, tomato and basil salad
Spaghetti vongole (clams)
Zabaglione

FRENCH
Moules marinière
Coq au vin; new potatoes; green vegetables
Crème caramel or sorbet

Fresh asparagus with melted butter
Sole bonne femme; new potatoes;
French beans
Petit pots au chocolat or chocolate mousse

MEXICAN
Tortilla chips with salsa dip
Chicken enchiladas; salad
2 margaritas (instead of dessert)

GREEK
Avgolemono soup
Souvlakia; tzatziki; salad; 1 piece bread
Fresh fruit and Greek yogurt

UK
Roast vegetable salad
Chargrilled salmon with coriander and lime; couscous
Fruit fool or lemon tart

UK (traditional)
Tomato soup; 1 small roll
225g grilled steak; baked potato; salad
Ice cream with chocolate sauce

Tips for minimising calorie intake when dining out

- Book your table for as early as you can – the later you leave it, the hungrier you will be and the more inclined to nibble on bread, crisps, etc.
- Say 'no' to butter and dressings as far as possible.
- If, after your main course, you aren't hungry, order one dessert for every two people and share – the taste is what you want, not the calories!
- Cheeseboard is usually much higher in calories than many desserts, so avoid it.
- Fresh fruit, when available, is the best dessert of all.

Where to eat

A look at the pros and cons of different types of restaurant.

Indian

- **Pros** Much traditional Indian fare is vegetarian with plenty of pulses such as chickpeas and lentils. High on taste – therefore you are likely to feel satisfied on not too many calories. Go for vegetable curries, pulse curries, tandoori dishes, plain or pilau rice, chapati, fresh fruit. Have small portions only of lentil or chickpea dahl, as they tend to be high in added oil.
- **Cons** Meat curries (and that includes chicken ones when the skin has been left on) may be very high in fat and saturated fat. Look out for liquid fat swimming on top of your curry dish. Some Indian curries include coconut which is very high fat, or cream, also high in fat. Korma and masala curries tend to be highest in cream. The typical deep-fried starters and accompaniments, such as bhajis and samosas, are very high in calories, and naan breads are also high in fat and calories. Although

poppadoms are deep-fried they tend not to absorb so much fat and as they weigh so little, won't do so much damage to your diet. But limit them to one or two.

Thai

- **Pros** Similar to Indian. Typical Thai food is very hot because of liberal use of chilli – a known metabolism booster. Go for soups, quick-cook 'sizzles' and stir-fries, chicken and vegetarian dishes, chilli prawns or crab.
- **Cons** Very strong on coconut cream and milk so try to pick dishes which don't contain these. Desserts are a waistline disaster – deep-fried bananas in batter with toffee sauce and coconut cream should be avoided!

Chinese

- **Pros** Very little red meat and no dairy produce; high on low-fat fish, lean pork, chicken, tofu, beansprouts and vegetables. Again, high on taste and if you use chopsticks you won't eat too quickly! Go for soups, stir-fries, dry-cooked spare ribs and steamed dishes, plain rice and fruit dessert. Chop sueys and chow mein aren't too bad as a main course choice either.
- **Cons** Can be high on fat if you pick the 'special-fried' dishes such as egg-fried rice, crispy-fried noodles, pork in batter, and so on. 'Wet' spare ribs will be very high in calories, as will spring rolls, deep-fried dumplings, and any braised dish which comes swimming in cooking oil.

Italian

- **Pros** Often high on salad, vegetables and fruit. A reasonably low-calorie meal can be found at almost all Italian restaurants. For starters choose melon, figs, Parma ham, artichokes, seafood salad. Good main courses for slimmers include pasta with seafood or tomato sauce, chicken cacciatore, veal, calf's liver, calamari. Best desserts are granita (sorbet-like), fresh fruit, zabaglione, baked peaches.

- **Cons** Many high-fat, high-calorie items also to be found on the menu. These include pasta starters, pasta main courses with cream/cheese/meat sauces, particularly carbonara, Bolognese, lasagne and cannelloni; risottos, which tend to be much higher in fat than you would think; and rich creamy desserts such as tiramisu and real dairy ice creams.

French

- **Pros** Can be good for fish and shellfish; soups and steaks, but much traditional French cuisine tends to be high in fat and rich sauces so watch out. Good starters include asparagus (eating only a small amount of butter); artichokes; snails; mussels. For a main course, choose plainly cooked fish, fish stew, steak, noisettes of lamb or pork tenderloin. Not much choice of low-calorie desserts – pears in wine or fresh fruit are probably best bets. Southern French restaurants may offer a better choice of dishes containing more vegetables and less saturated fat – items such as tuna with ratatouille are reasonable bets if offered. Go for potatoes Lyonnaise or new potatoes, and peas with lettuce.
- **Cons** May offer too many cream- and butter-rich sauces and dishes. For starters, avoid pâté, coquilles St Jacques, and most soups. French casseroles are typically made with fatty bacon and a lot of oil. Fish often comes in creamy sauce – avoid 'meunière' or 'bonne femme'. Avoid sliced potatoes baked in cream (dauphinoise). Desserts are mostly high in fat – avoid crème brûlée, chocolate mousse, profiteroles and tarte tatin.

Greek

- **Pros** High in salads, lean meat, plenty of grills and fish available. Go for feta salad starters or tzatziki and pitta; for main course try pork, chicken or lamb kebabs, grilled fish, klefarico (roast lamb), dolmades (stuffed vine leaves) with bread and side salads; fresh fruit or Greek yogurt and honey for dessert.
- **Cons** Some dishes can be very high in fat – avoid taramasalata as a starter; moussaka, spinach and cheese pie, or stifado (a beef stew that can be very oily). Desserts are mostly extremely sweet and rich and fatty. Avoid baklava and halva.

Japanese

- **Pros** Generally light on fat and a good bet for slimmers. High on fish, rice, vegetables.
- **Cons** Few.

Tips on reducing your alcohol intake

Many a big belly has been blamed on beer, and although the 'beer gut' is a bit of a misnomer (as your stomach can get fat through overeating as well as overindulging in alcohol) it is quite true that alcohol *is* fattening and is largely surplus to our nutritional requirements. One gram of alcohol contains 7 calories (as opposed to 4 for protein and 3.75 for carbohydrates). Only fat is more fattening, at 9 calories a gram. Though there are trace minerals and vitamins in some alcoholic drinks (e.g. dark beers) you would need to take in vast quantities for the nutritional aspect to be significant. Therefore it is a good idea to limit your intake when you are trying to lose weight.

Although in moderation it can be quite good for your health (a moderate intake of wine and beer has been shown to help protect against heart disease, atherosclerosis and so on), it is also a good idea to keep intake low if you want to live a long and healthy life. Just as importantly, too much alcohol can wreck your business life as well.

So, for reasons of size and health, I have limited the amount of alcohol you are supposed to drink on the Business Plan to an absolute maximum of 250 calories' worth a day – that is about half a bottle of wine or just over two halves of beer or lager. On **BASIC** days, you should be having no more than one glass if your evening meal allows it (see pages 120–2).

Yet alcohol seems such an ingrained part of many people's daily business lives. The tips below will, I hope, help you to moderate your intake. If you feel that your career or your business depends upon your alcohol consumption – think again.

TIPS for cutting back

- If you like white wine, mix it half and half with soda water or sparkling mineral water.
- Alternate each alcoholic drink you take with a non-alcoholic one.
- Choose low-alcohol versions of wine, beer, cider.
- Recognise the triggers that make you drink alcohol and try to find ways of changing them, e.g. you always have a drink when you get home in the evening. Change your routine slightly and have a bath or a walk round the garden when you get in.
- Take some exercise. All research shows that people who exercise really do find that their taste and capacity for alcohol diminishes.
- Don't drink before a meal; you will always drink more before a meal than during or after.
- Have water to quench your thirst before beginning on any alcohol; it is easy to quaff light wine or beer just to stem thirst when water would do the job better.

- Don't have salty snacks such as peanuts and crisps when you are in a pub or wine bar or in someone's home. These increase thirst and have been shown to make people drink more.
- Cut out lunchtime drinking altogether – many people these days have a rule not to drink until evening and no one will think you are being ridiculous if you stick to water at meetings and when socialising earlier in the day.
- Set a 'drink time' in the evening, before and after which you know you won't drink. If you enjoy wine with your evening meal, your drink time could be between 8pm and 9pm, for instance.
- If at a social gathering, don't hold your glass – put it down between sips. You will drink at half the speed.
- If you think you regularly drink too much, try to analyse reasons for this, apart from ones of habit. If you have life problems, try to sort these out so that you don't resort to alcohol as a comfort.
- Tell your partner that you are going to cut down on alcohol and enlist their help.
- Work out how much money you will save over the course of a year by halving your alcohol intake, or by giving it up altogether.
- Write a list of all the things you'd like to do with the money saved – pick one or more and do them.

Entertaining at home

If you have to do a lot of entertaining at home, there is no need to go over the top with a lot of high-fat, high-cream dishes. These days very many people you are likely to entertain actually prefer lighter dishes that rely for their taste on good quality basic produce, herbs, spices and so on.

I've put together five delicious three-course menus here, all of which come to around 1,000 calories each. These fit in well with the 1,000-calorie guidelines for your **BIG EVENING** days.

If you want to drink alcohol with your meal, limit it to 1–2 glasses or have alcohol instead of a dessert, in which case you can have about half a bottle, and follow the tips on pages 129–30 for limiting your intake on social occasions.

Other recipes in this book are also suitable for entertaining. Have a look at the various recipe sections and put together some more ideas for yourself. The Meat-Free Plan contains a variety of non-meat recipes; the Fast Food Plan has ideas for producing good main courses when you are in a hurry; the Family Plan contains some lower-cost menus and the Sweet-tooth Plan has a recipe section containing many mouth-watering desserts.

Tips for entertaining

- Light starters include anything based on fruit, vegetables or salads. A perfect melon; a light vegetable soup; a plate of fresh asparagus; a few creamy avocado slices mixed with crisp lettuce leaves and drizzled with balsamic vinegar – these have a quarter the calories of traditional starters such as prawn cocktails, creamed soups, high saturated-fat meat pâtés, and so on.
- You could also skip a traditional starter and simply offer your guests a beautiful plateful of crudités such as strips of red pepper, carrot, yellow pepper, spring onions and so on with a dip of garlicky tzatziki (natural bio yogurt mixed with crushed garlic and chopped cucumber and seasoned well) or of low-fat mayonnaise mixed half and half with yogurt and enlivened with chopped herbs or chilli sauce or curry powder.

- Offer this over a welcome drink in the sitting room or kitchen before sitting down to dine and this also gets over the problem of whether or not to offer all those fattening pre-dinner nibbles like nuts and crisps. This way, you don't need to!
- If you have offered a starter as well as a main course, it is nowadays perfectly acceptable to forget desserts as such and simply offer a lovely bowl of fruit as a table centrepiece after the main course and offer a cheeseboard with it for those who are still hungry. This saves your precious time as well.
- If your dinner table has a mix of guests who are watching their weight and others who are 16-stone rugby forwards or similar with large appetites, simply have a good bread basket so that they can help themselves throughout the meal, and cook extra of the carbohydrate portion of your main course – potatoes, rice, pasta, couscous or whatever. Those extras plus the cheeseboard mentioned above will ensure no one needs to go home hungry.

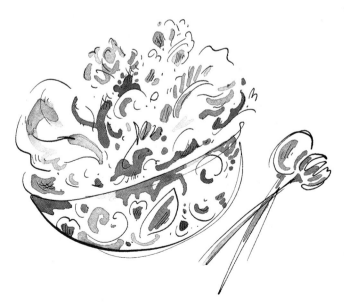

Five Three-course Menus for Entertaining

Each of these is 1,000 calories in total or less.

MENU 1

Suitable for: *Summer; demi-vegetarians; whole menu easy.*

Watercress soup*
Spiced Creamy Salmon with Lentils*
Couscous
Side salad
Individual Summer Puddings*
Greek yogurt

MENU 2

Suitable for: *Autumn or winter; quick and easy starter and dessert; easy main course.*

Hot Bacon, Garlic and Chicken Liver Salad*
Venison and Guinea Fowl Casserole*
Bulghar Wheat
Broccoli
Cabbage
Fruit Kebabs with Butter and Honey Sauce*

MENU 3

Suitable for: *Any season; fairly quick to prepare; fairly easy starter, easy main course, very easy dessert.*

Mediterranean Stuffed Tomatoes with Mozzarella*
Coq au Vin Blanc*
New potatoes
Mangetout
Spinach
Flambéed Pineapple and Banana*

MENU 4

Suitable for: *Particularly summer, but can be easily adapted for any season; no red meat; quick and easy starter and dessert.*

Artichoke and Grilled Red Pepper Salad*
Paella*
Peach Melba Layer*

MENU 5

Suitable for: *Spring or summer; demi-vegetarians; whole menu quick and easy.*

Melon, Prawn and Avocado Salad*
Tagliatelle with Smoked Salmon and Broccoli*
Dipping Fruits and Chocolate Sauce*

* SEE RECIPE SECTION, PAGES 133–9.

15 RECIPES FOR ENTERTAINING

MENU 1

WATERCRESS SOUP

Serves 4
155 calories and 2.5g fat per portion

450g old potatoes
600ml vegetable stock
2 bunches fresh watercress
400ml skimmed milk
1 medium onion, chopped
Salt and black pepper
2 tablespoons single cream

Peel the potatoes, chop them into fairly small chunks and put in a saucepan with the stock. Bring to a simmer. Pick over the watercress and remove any tough stalks or yellow leaves. Save four sprigs for garnish, if liked. Add to the pan with the milk, onion and seasoning and simmer, covered, for about 20 minutes.

Allow to cool a little, then blend in an electric blender until smooth but not overprocessed. Return to the saucepan to heat through again. Before serving, check seasoning. To serve, stir a little cream into the top of each portion of soup and garnish with the reserved watercress sprigs.

SPICED CREAMY SALMON WITH LENTILS

Serves 4
470 calories and 23g fat per portion

1 tablespoon sunflower oil
1 onion, finely chopped
1 clove garlic, crushed
1 level tablespoon garam masala
1 × 400g can brown lentils, drained
1 × 400g can chopped tomatoes with chilli
150ml fish stock
Salt and black pepper
4 × 125g salmon fillets
2 tablespoons half-fat crème fraîche

Heat the oil in a large lidded non-stick frying pan and add the onion and garlic; cook for a few minutes, stirring occasionally. Add the garam masala and stir for another minute, then add the lentils, tomatoes, stock and seasoning to taste, and stir to combine everything. Simmer gently, uncovered, for 15 minutes, stirring now and then. Add the salmon fillets to the pan and simmer, covered, for another few minutes depending upon the thickness of the fillets (5–10 minutes). When cooked, remove the salmon fillets, add the crème fraîche to the pan and stir in. Place the salmon fillets on the bed of spiced creamy lentils. Serve with 150g (dry weight) couscous, reconstituted (for four), plus a side salad. This will add approx. 150 calories per portion.

INDIVIDUAL SUMMER PUDDINGS

Serves 4
175 calories and 1.5g fat per portion

225g blackcurrants

125g redcurrants

325g raspberries

6 slices of white bread from a large sliced loaf

2 rounded tablespoons fructose

Heat the fruits in a saucepan with a very little water and simmer gently for a few minutes until the blackcurrants are beginning to burst and there is plenty of juice in the pan.

Meanwhile, cut the crusts off the bread and quarter each slice. When the fruit is ready stir in the fructose (see below). Divide half the bread quarters between four glass dessert dishes, then spoon over half the fruit with its juice. Make another similar layer, spooning all the juice in the pan over the dishes so that the bread is covered. Chill for an hour or two before serving. Serve with 1 tablespoon of full-fat Greek yogurt each, which will add about 20 calories per portion to the dessert.

NOTE *Fructose is fruit sugar, which is sweeter than ordinary sugar and so you need to use less. It goes particularly well with fruit desserts such as this.*

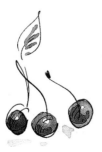

MENU 2

HOT BACON, GARLIC AND CHICKEN LIVER SALAD

Serves 4
340 calories and 18g fat per portion

1 × 200g pack mixed salad leaves with herbs

2 × 25g slices bread, crusts removed

3 tablespoons olive oil

2 cloves garlic, peeled and crushed

100g extra-lean unsmoked back bacon, cut into strips

1 tablespoon red wine vinegar

1 teaspoon wholegrain mustard

1 level teaspoon brown caster sugar

Salt and black pepper

140g French bread

12 chicken livers, halved, soaked in milk for 30 minutes, then drained

Arrange the salad leaves in four serving bowls. Brush the slices of bread with a little of the olive oil, then rub with a little of the garlic; cut the bread into bite-sized squares and bake in the oven at 190°C/375°F/Gas 5 until golden and crisp. Take out and reserve.

Heat 1 dessertspoon of the remaining oil in a non-stick frying pan and fry the bacon until it is crisp and golden. Remove with a slotted spoon and reserve, leaving the oil in the pan.

Meanwhile, make a salad dressing by combining the remaining olive oil with the vinegar, mustard, sugar and seasoning and shake well in a screw-top jar. Cut the French bread into four slices.

Reheat the oil in the frying pan and stir-fry the chicken livers, adding the garlic after a minute or so. The livers will take only two minutes to cook. Return the bacon to the pan for the last 30 seconds of cooking time and, just before serving, pour the salad dressing into the pan too. Serve the salad leaves with the liver and bacon mixture lightly tossed in and with the croûtons sprinkled on top. Serve with the French bread.

VENISON AND GUINEA FOWL CASSEROLE

Serves 4
330 calories and 11.5g fat per portion

1 tablespoon olive oil

250g cubed venison

4 breasts guinea fowl, skin removed and each cut into 3

16 small shallots, peeled

1 large green pepper, deseeded and sliced

2 cloves garlic, peeled and chopped

1 bay leaf

Sprig fresh thyme or use 1 teaspoon dried thyme

6 juniper berries if available

1 tablespoon plain flour

3 tablespoons brandy

100ml red wine

1 rounded tablespoon tomato purée

Approx. 150ml beef stock

Salt and black pepper

225g mushrooms, halved if small, otherwise sliced

Heat the oil in a lidded flameproof casserole and add the venison pieces and the guinea fowl. Don't stir or turn for two minutes until the undersides are golden, otherwise the meat may stick. Turn and brown the other sides, then remove the meat from the casserole and reserve. Add the shallots to the pan and sauté until tinged with gold, then add the green pepper and garlic and stir for 2–3 minutes. Add all the rest of the ingredients (which should all be cool, otherwise the flour may not mix in smoothly) except the mushrooms. Stir well, return the meat to the pan, bring to a simmer, cover and cook for 1½ hours.

Stir the mushrooms into the casserole and cook for a further 20 minutes. Check the seasoning and serve with 150g (dry weight) bulghar wheat, reconstituted (for four), plus broccoli and cabbage. This will add approx. 170 calories per portion.

FRUIT KEBABS WITH BUTTER AND HONEY SAUCE

Serves 4
140 calories and 2.5g fat per portion

1 mango

2 medium bananas

4 pineapple slices, quartered, or 200g pineapple chunks, drained

15g half-fat Anchor butter, melted

1 tablespoon runny honey

1 dessertspoon lemon juice

4 tablespoons half-fat crème fraîche

Peel and stone the mango and cut into 12 chunks. Peel the bananas and cut into 8 chunks. Thread the mango, banana and pineapple pieces on to four kebab skewers and brush with a little of the half-fat butter. Grill under a hot heat, turning from time to time, for a few minutes until softened.

Meanwhile, in a small saucepan, heat the rest of the butter, the honey and lemon juice and beat to combine. Baste the kebabs with a little of this mixture just before the end of cooking, then serve the kebabs with the honey sauce poured over and with 1 tablespoon of the crème fraîche each.

NOTE If you have any juice from the mango you can pour that into the sauce as well.

MENU 3

MEDITERRANEAN STUFFED TOMATOES WITH MOZZARELLA

Serves 4
237 calories and 12g per portion

2 beef tomatoes (approx. 200g each)

Salt

2 large cloves garlic, peeled

1 pot fresh basil leaves

40g fresh Parmesan cheese, grated

2 medium tomatoes, skinned, deseeded and chopped

1 tablespoon olive oil

1 level tablespoon pine nuts

100g half-fat mozzarella cheese

1 heaped tablespoon stale breadcrumbs

4 × 25g slices French or ciabatta bread

Halve the beef tomatoes horizontally and scoop out the seeds, then sprinkle them with a little salt. Using a pestle and mortar, pound the garlic with a little more salt, then pound in the basil and Parmesan; add the chopped tomatoes and pound again, then the olive oil and mix again. Finally, stir in the pine nuts but don't pound them. Fill the tomato cavities with the basil–tomato stuffing. Slice the mozzarella into four and top each tomato half with a slice, then sprinkle the stale breadcrumbs on top. At this stage you can leave the tomatoes for a while if necessary.

Half an hour before you want to serve them, preheat the oven to 200°C/400°F/Gas 6, then cook the tomatoes on a baking sheet for 15 minutes or so, until the tops are golden; serve with the slices of bread.

COQ AU VIN BLANC

Serves 4
435 calories and 13.5g fat per portion

8 medium bone-in chicken thigh pieces, skin removed

1 rounded tablespoon plain flour

Salt and black pepper

1½ tablespoons olive oil

16 small shallots, peeled

110g lean unsmoked gammon, cut into strips

3 tablespoons brandy

300ml dry white wine

250ml chicken stock

2 cloves garlic, peeled and crushed

1 bouquet garni

75g bread

225g chestnut mushrooms, halved or sliced

Fresh parsley, finely chopped

Coat the chicken pieces with the flour and seasoning (if you put everything into a large plastic bag and shake well, this is done quickly). Heat the oil in a large flameproof casserole or good quality large lidded non-stick frying pan, and add the shallots. Over a medium high heat, cook them for a few minutes, turning occasionally, until lightly golden. Remove with a slotted spoon and reserve. Add the chicken pieces and gammon and cook over a high heat until lightly golden, turning once. Pour the brandy around the chicken and set it alight, standing well back (if you wish, this bit is optional). When the flames have died down, return the shallots to the pan along with the wine, stock, garlic, bouquet garni and any flour that remains from coating the chicken. Stir well, cover and simmer for 1 hour.

Meanwhile, chop the bread roughly, lay it on a baking tray and bake at 180°C/375°F/Gas 5 or until golden and crisp.

When the chicken is ready, add the mushrooms and simmer again for 15 minutes. To finish, remove the bouquet garni, check the seasoning and stir in the parsley. Sprinkle the bread over the top and serve with potatoes and vegetables.

NOTE *If the sauce needs thickening further, remove the chicken, etc. with a slotted spoon and boil the remaining liquid in the casserole for a few minutes until reduced.*

FLAMBÉED PINEAPPLE AND BANANA

Serves 4
177 calories and 4g fat per portion

15g half-fat Anchor butter

300g ready-prepared fresh pineapple chunks, drained and dried and juice reserved

2 medium bananas, barely ripe

1 tablespoon caster sugar

1 tablespoon rum

4 scoops Too Good to be True iced dessert, vanilla

Heat the butter in a non-stick frying pan and when bubbling, add the pineapple chunks and stir for a minute. Peel the bananas and cut each into four pieces and add to the pan. Cook over a medium heat for several minutes until the fruit begins to turn golden. Add the sugar and stir well for another minute. Add the rum and set it alight. When the flames die down, add a little pineapple juice to the pan, stir quickly and divide the fruit between four serving dishes and serve with the iced dessert.

MENU 4

ARTICHOKE AND GRILLED RED PEPPER SALAD

Serves 4
120 calories and 8g fat per portion

2 large red peppers, halved and deseeded

2 tablespoons olive oil

2 small Little Gem lettuces

8 canned artichoke hearts, well drained

1 tablespoon red wine vinegar

1 teaspoon wholegrain mustard

1 level teaspoon caster sugar

Salt and black pepper

8 anchovy fillets

Heat the grill, brush the peppers with a little of the olive oil and grill until the edges are beginning to blacken.

Meanwhile, cut each lettuce into eight wedges and divide between four serving plates, then arrange the artichoke hearts among the lettuce wedges. When the peppers are ready, cut into strips and arrange on the salads.

Shake together the remaining olive oil, vinegar, mustard, sugar and seasoning and pour over the salads, then top with the anchovy fillets.

PAELLA

Serves 4
630 calories and 12g fat per portion

3 × 125g chicken breast fillets, skin removed

2 plum tomatoes, drained

1 pack saffron threads

2 tablespoons olive oil

1 large green pepper, deseeded and chopped

1 medium onion, chopped

1 teaspoon paprika

800ml chicken stock

275g long-grain rice

110g petit pois

Salt and black pepper

20 mussels in their shells, ready prepared

200g peeled prawns

8 large unshelled cooked prawns to garnish

Cut each chicken breast into four, chop the tomatoes and soak the saffron threads in a little water. Heat the oil in a very large non-stick frying pan or paella pan (use two pans if necessary) and sauté the chicken and onion until golden. Add the tomatoes, peppers, onion and saffron plus soaking water, paprika and a little of the stock and simmer for 15 minutes. Add the rice, peas and some more stock and seasoning and stir well. Bring back to a simmer and cook gently until the rice is tender, adding more stock as necessary. When the rice is cooked, stir in the mussels and peeled prawns and warm through. When the mussels open, the paella is ready. Serve garnished with the unshelled prawns.

NOTE *If you can find uncooked unshelled prawns, use them instead of the cooked ones. Add about 5 minutes before the end of cooking time.*

PEACH MELBA LAYER

Serves 4
257 calories and 8g fat per portion

150g raspberries

1 dessertspoon icing sugar

25ml framboise liqueur

2 ripe peaches or nectarines, peeled, stoned and sliced

4 meringue nests, crumbled

4 scoops Too Good to be True vanilla iced dessert, allowed to soften

100g Delight Whipping Cream Alternative, whipped

1 tablespoon chopped mixed nuts

Using an electric blender, purée the raspberries with the sugar and liqueur. Using four glass serving dishes or stemmed glasses, layer the desserts as follows, dividing the ingredients evenly between the glasses: peaches, meringue, ice cream dessert, raspberry sauce, whipped cream, nuts. Serve immediately.

NOTE *If you don't want to use framboise liqueur, use a tablespoon of peach or similar juice instead.*

MENU 5

MELON, PRAWN AND AVOCADO SALAD

Serves 4
240 calories and 19.5g fat per portion

1 tablespoon lime juice

1 pinch saffron

1 small cantaloupe melon (about 400g unprepared weight, about 325g melon flesh)

2 tablespoons walnut oil

Salt and black pepper

2 small ripe avocados

225g peeled prawns, preferably fresh and good quality

4 unpeeled prawns

Mix together the lime juice and saffron and leave for half an hour. Ball the melon or cut it into bite-sized chunks. Mix together the oil, lime juice mixture and seasoning. Peel, halve and stone the avocados and slice horizontally, then halve each slice so you have bite-sized pieces. In a bowl, combine all these ingredients with the peeled prawns. Divide between four glass serving dishes or glasses and top with a whole prawn. Chill to serve.

TAGLIATELLE WITH SMOKED SALMON AND BROCCOLI

Serves 4
511 calories and 15.5g fat per portion

300g (dry weight) tagliatelle

200g broccoli florets

100g petit pois

15g butter (1 tablespoon)

4 shallots, finely chopped

2 tablespoons dry white wine

200ml half-fat crème fraîche

A little fish, chicken or vegetable stock

1 level tablespoon chopped dill plus dill leaves
    for garnish

250g good quality smoked salmon, cut into strips

Cook the pasta in a large pan of boiling salted water for 12 minutes or according to pack instructions; drain.

Meanwhile, boil the broccoli and peas in two pans until just cooked but still firm. Drain and reserve. When the pasta is half cooked, heat the butter in a non-stick frying pan and sauté the shallots until

softened and transparent. Add the wine and stir for a minute. Add the crème fraîche and stir, adding a little stock until you have the consistency of single cream. Add the chopped dill. Tip the cooked, drained pasta into serving bowls, stir in the vegetables, smoked salmon and cream sauce and serve immediately, garnished with extra dill, if you like.

DIPPING FRUITS AND CHOCOLATE SAUCE

Serves 4
190 calories and 9g fat per portion

150g large strawberries, hulled and quartered

2 peaches or nectarines, stoned and cut into slices

150g fresh pineapple chunks

100g dark good quality chocolate

25ml single cream

Divide the fruits between four serving plates or arrange on one big platter. Break the chocolate into a small heatproof bowl and melt over a pan of simmering water. Make sure that the bowl doesn't touch the water and that the bowl fits tightly into the pan so that steam cannot escape, otherwise the chocolate may curdle.

When the chocolate is melted, stir in the cream to combine. Serve immediately so that your guests can dip the fruit into the chocolate sauce.

NOTE *Alternatively, you could pour the sauce over the fruits on each plate and the dessert could be eaten with spoons.*

CASE HISTORY

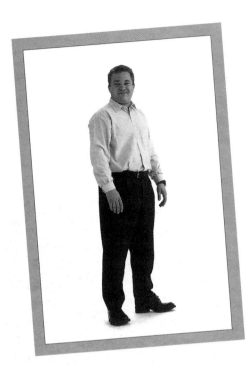

GARETH DIXON

AGE: **28**

STATUS: **Married; no children**

OCCUPATION: **Has own marketing consultancy**

HEIGHT: **5 ft 4 ins**

START WEIGHT: **12 st 13 lb**

WEIGHT AFTER SIX WEEKS: **12 st**

STARTING BMI: **32**

BMI AFTER SIX WEEKS: **29.8**

STARTING STATISTICS: **Chest – 39½ Waist – 37½**

STATISTICS AFTER SIX WEEKS: **Chest – 38 Waist – 34**

Like many young men, Gareth began to pile on weight after he left school and gave up sport – rugby, in his case. At university, his lifestyle consisted of 'very little exercise, lots of drinking and eating bad food!' Then came the world of business, entertaining clients and too much rich food and more drink.

By the time I met Gareth he weighed nearly 13 stone with Body Mass Index of 32, meaning he was clinically obese before the age of 30.

'When I saw your advert for people who wanted to lose weight, I was attracted because I needed an independent person telling me what to do – not my wife Kirsten, as I would feel I was being nagged! Although I carry my weight well, I wanted to feel healthier, get rid of my big, bloated tummy, my fat face and my double chin, which I hate. And I wanted to get into clothes that suit my height, not my width.

'I knew I was overweight at a very early age, and the thought of perhaps becoming a father, and not wanting to be fat and unfit, was my main motivation.'

I analysed Gareth's pre-plan eating diary and it reminded me of *Men Behaving Badly* – lots of beer, wine, red meat every day, take-aways, huge baguettes filled with beef – no fruit, no salad . . . and so on!

'I really do want to eat more healthily, though,' said Gareth. 'Just tell me what I have to do!' As Gareth leads the typical life of a busy businessman, we naturally put him on the Business Plan.

'I started eating fruit (a first for me) and also gave myself time for proper breakfast. After the first two or three days, which were very hard, I found the programme great.

'We enjoyed cooking the recipes, especially pasta dishes and rice, and I didn't find eating out too much of a problem once I knew the kind of dishes I had to stick to. Kirsten was very supportive with lots of encouragement.

'I have a bad back due to an old rugby injury so I was wary about exercise, but Sarah showed me how to do abdominals without risk to the back, and I began going out running for 20 minutes, two or three times a week, sometimes for longer. As this became noticeably easier, I felt great. Now I feel more alert at home and more energetic in the evenings when I get home from work. I'm much happier mentally – I felt fantastic when I saw the weight start to come off and other people started noticing – and feel better physically.

'Ideally I want to lose some more weight and I know now that it is the combination of diet and exercise that will help me get slim and keep it off. I still enjoy drinking, but much less now. I say one thing to being nearly 13 stone and unfit – *never again*!'

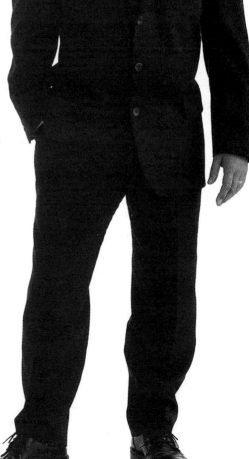

Suit Gareth's own, Grattan Pierre Cardin shirt and tie

the family plan

Few people start out in life fat. Indeed, by the time we reach adulthood only 8 per cent of us are, officially, carrying too much weight. But that figure begins to rise as soon as we hit the twenties and by the time we are 30-plus we stand a 40 per cent chance of being clinically overweight or obese.

I believe that the major reason for this is not greed or a genetic tendency to get fat but simply that the way we live makes us fat. A busy career can do it – a problem shared by both men and women – but by far the most common factor affecting women in their late twenties, thirties and forties is family life.

I say 'women' because all surveys show even if the female partner/wife/mother works, she often still runs the kitchen and all that entails.

So this Family Plan is unashamedly aimed mostly at women. If you happen to be male and looking after the family food – it will work for you too!

Food for thought

But just why is family life so bad for the waistline? If you look at the reasons, then get them fixed firmly in your mind, it will help you to overcome them.

Even if there are no children around yet, the pounds can begin creeping on as soon as the

honeymoon begins, or you start living together. Because women are, generally, shorter than men, they need to eat less to maintain a reasonable body weight. Single and independent, most women realise this and quite naturally follow a regime that helps them to do just that.

But the minute you begin living with a man, all that common sense seems to vanish. He's hungry – you cook him a suitable man-sized meal, which of course you have to share with him. He's hungry and you won't cook him a meal . . . he cooks it himself and expects you to share it with him, every last drop of saturated fat included, dishing you out a huge portion. He's hungry and you're out – he eats up everything he can find in the refrigerator, including what you'd planned to eat yourself – so you end up with something more fattening. You have an argument – and make it up by preparing him a special three-course meal. You are fed up arguing over who cooks dinner – so you end up eating out. You have an argument – you eat a pack of biscuits for comfort.

Now there's someone to share meals with, it's nice to include a bottle of wine at night. You didn't used to bother with lunch at weekends but now you've got into the habit of it. He enjoys a fry-up at weekend breakfast time, too – and it smells so good, you eat it as well.

And so on. And so on. When you have a partner, food is no longer just sustenance that you shop for and prepare and eat in the shortest time possible. It tends to fulfil a different function in your life together – and the result is weight on you. (And probably him, as well.)

Then when you have children, the problems are compounded. You're not eating for two (you and your partner), but three, or four or more. It certainly isn't just the pregnancies that put weight on you, but the children.

There are even more meals to prepare (often parents and children eat separately) and more time spent around food, and this encourages a natural tendency to pick. The worst time of day for many a mother is the children's teatime when she is ravenous after work and before her own meal. How many chips get eaten while you're dishing out the kids' meals? How many more get eaten when they leave some on their plates? We all know the answer to that.

Budgeting may also be a factor, with low-cost foods the only option. How many women have said to me that they can't lose weight because they can't afford 'slimming foods'? (A myth I aim to dispel.)

Once the kids become teenagers, and are eating with you now, you find many become ravenous, especially boys, so they demand huge platefuls of highly dense food – just the sort of thing you would ideally like to cut back on.

And even when the kids have left home, if your partner has still managed to hang on in there and keep your affection, your eating life still isn't your own. The ultimate unfair insult is the one horrible husbands frequently use on their wives: You're fat; why don't you do something about it? Knowing what I know now about food and family life, if my husband ever said that to me, I think I'd kill him!

Solutions

There is no one simple solution to all these scenarios – but knowing that they exist and becoming aware of them on a day-to-day basis is a big step towards getting them under control.

The following pages offer my best tips for eating for weight control within family life; and the diet plan and the family-friendly recipes that follow aim to provide you with the ammunition to see your resolutions through.

Top 10 Tips for Slimming Within the Family

- Redevelop your sense of self. This doesn't exactly mean being selfish – but be a bit less selfless when it comes to what food you buy and what you prepare. When you shop, make sure to include plenty of the things that *you* like and that will help you stick to a slimming plan. These are not necessarily all expensive things (see below). If you have children who are still very young, it is an excellent policy to get them eating healthily. Although young children shouldn't be given a very low-fat wholefood diet (they should be given whole milk; white bread may be preferable at least some of the time for its calcium content; and if underweight they should be given more energy-dense foods like potatoes – chips, even – cheese and bread), neither do they need lots of sweets; heavy, sickly desserts; salty, fatty snacks; fatty meat or sugary drinks. Avoid buying these things regularly right from the start.

- Most children over the age of four have lunch away from home – either a packed lunch or in a school cafeteria. If packed is an option, go for it. This is your main opportunity to provide them with the calories and nutrients they need, while avoiding the calories yourself. It is also a good time to let them have their own favourite things, within the bounds of what we've discussed above. There is no harm in giving any child, unless he is obese, plenty of sandwiches, cake (preferably fruit cake, malt loaf, or something not too sugary or artificial), milk, even some chocolate. Nuts and seeds are good for children over five who aren't allergic to them. Add a piece of fruit and you have a good calorific meal.

- All children and teenagers, unless fat, will benefit from a snack when they come in from school or college. Let them eat bread, spread and Marmite or jam; or teacakes or scones or crumpets. If hungry teens have a good mid-afternoon snack they will be happy with a less calorific meal when you all eat. When it is time for small children's tea, try to plan ahead and prepare things like casseroles which you won't be so tempted to 'steal'. Have a snack for yourself handy when preparing tea or, indeed, any meal, for others that you won't be eating yourself – fruit or crudités and a low-fat dip, such as those by Iceland, or yogurt and cucumber. Try to exercise portion control for children so you don't get leftovers. If you do, give them to the dog or cat or put them straight in the bin.

- Older children and/or a partner who will be eating the same meal as you in the evening needn't be a problem. The meals and recipes in this plan show you that you can all eat the same thing. Give them bigger portions, and add to what they eat with extra carbohydrates – bread, potatoes, pasta, rice, etc. They can have a dollop of butter on their vegetables or baked potato, and they can also have a dessert, e.g. banana and custard, fruit and cream, yogurt.

- Don't say you're on a slimming diet; say you are going to begin eating more healthily (if necessary say your doctor has told you to). Men and children hate the idea of 'slimming' and 'slimming foods'. Quite right too, really – there is no need to think like this. I have had dozens of successful slimmers saying to me that their husbands, or friends who come round to dinner, have been amazed when they have found out that what they are eating is suitable for slimmers.

- Do plan ahead. I'd say weekly forward thinking will be vital to the success of your slimming effort. A little time spent once a week planning your week's menus will save much time in the shop and hassle in the kitchen, and will save all those high-calorie snacks and nibbles that are popped in your mouth because you can't find a suitable alternative. Write lists before you shop and try to avoid shopping with children who will undoubtedly persuade you to buy things that may be better left on the shelf.

- Be fully aware of what you are eating and why. Go back to our introduction and my long list of occasions when you have probably been eating for the wrong reasons, and, every week, try to give your body only what it needs, not a lot of unnecessary food. Again – be selfish. Eventually you will find you can stop yourself from eating unless you are hungry and genuinely need the food. Also remember that weight gain is not just caused by what you eat at the meal table, but what you eat in between and out of the home – snacks.

- Start some foolproof strategies to prevent the other members of the family sabotaging your efforts. By this I mean take steps to prevent them pinching your own private food or drinks. Keep a large lidded container in the refrigerator with your name on it for items you may use for breakfast or lunch – e.g. low-fat bio yogurts, fruit, lower-fat cheeses, carton soups, and so on.

- Special meals – we all have occasions when we want to produce something special. That's fine. These won't be that often, you can budget for them and there are plenty of ideas for three-course meals at home on page 132. If your partner or the kids want to cook you a meal, then at least you should have the chance to decide what you want, and then you can choose something that won't wreck your diet. If they cook on a regular basis, either copy out the recipes in this section or invest in some low-calorie cookbooks and let them choose. I've written several myself and they don't actually look much like 'diet' cookbooks, nor eat like them. If you do get faced with a huge plateful swimming in fat and a proud face determined to watch you eat every mouthful – eat it, but before the next time, remind him/them that you want to watch your intake of fat/sugar or whatever and again help by providing suitable recipes, or offering tips on shopping (e.g. buy extra-lean cuts of meat, lower-fat creams, and so on). If your partner likes you to eat out a lot, then turn to Chapter 7 for lots of information on making wise choices in the restaurant.

- But slimming food is too dear ... Actually, no it isn't. You don't have to buy out-of-season salads, fruits or vegetables, or veal or grouse or guinea fowl if you don't want to. There are always cheaper fruits and vegetables in season, and the low-calorie meats such as chicken, turkey, and some fishes, are not expensive. Cheapest of all are the 'good for you' carbohydrates such as bread, potatoes, pasta and rice – which all the family loves.

In this plan I have offered a few more expensive dishes but there is no need to choose anything costly at all if you don't want to. If you are cutting down on fattening items – perhaps sweet foods like biscuits, cakes, desserts – you will have more money to spare for the extra fruit and vegetables you will undoubtedly be buying.

What to do

- Read Chapters 1 and 2, and the introductory pages of this chapter, before beginning this plan!
- Each week of the diet has a separate page.
- Every day pick one Breakfast, one Lunch, one Main Meal and one Snack or Treat from the suggestions.
- In addition to these meals and snacks, you can have:

Unlimiteds

The following are unlimited on the plan:
- *Drinks* Water, mineral water, herbal teas, green tea, ordinary tea and coffee (with milk from allowance, no sugar), lemon juice, calorie-free soft drinks and mixers.
- *Foods* Salad greens, cucumber, onion, cress, leafy green vegetables, carrots.
- *Condiments* Fresh or dried herbs and spices, Worcestershire sauce, light soy sauce, tomato purée, passata, vinegar, oil-free French dressing and other calorie-free dressings, low-fat stock cubes.

Milk Allowance

A daily milk allowance of 250ml skimmed or 200ml semi-skimmed milk for use in tea or coffee or as a drink on its own. If not required, have one 125ml tub of natural low-fat yogurt. Milk for breakfast cereals is on top of this allowance.

Bread

When 'one slice bread' is mentioned within the plan, unless otherwise stated, this means one slice of bread from a large medium-cut loaf with a little low-fat spread. This can of course be toasted if liked.

Fruit

When 'I portion fruit' is mentioned, unless otherwise stated, this means one medium piece of fruit other than banana (e.g. apple, orange, nectarine) or 2 small fruits (e.g. plums, satsumas) or a medium bowlful small berry fruits (e.g. strawberries, raspberries), or 75g grapes or cherries; or a medium bowlful fresh fruit salad.

WEEK ONE

Notes

- Eat all you are allowed on the plan.
- Try to plan ahead.
- Read the instructions and the start of this chapter before you begin.

Breakfasts

- 40g All-Bran or 30g Just Right with 125ml skimmed milk and 1 portion fruit added, chopped as necessary, 4 pieces ready-to-eat dried apricot.
- 1 slice bread, 2 teaspoons low-sugar jam or marmalade; 1 large banana; 1 small glass unsweetened orange juice.
- 150ml low-fat natural bio yogurt; 25g muesli; 1 portion fruit; 1 dessertspoon sesame seeds.

Lunches

- Sandwich of 2 slices bread filled with 100g tuna in brine or water, drained, 1 dessertspoon Kraft Free Choice mayonnaise and salad items of choice; 1 portion fruit.
- Salad of 1 small cooked chicken portion plus large mixed salad and 4 tablespoons cold cooked rice or pasta mixed with oil-free French dressing and 4 pieces ready-to-eat dried apricot; Shape fruit fromage frais.
- Any take-away ready sandwich containing 300 calories or less (check label); 1 portion fruit.
- Half a 400g can baked beans on 1 slice toast; 1 large banana.
- 1 whole carton New Covent Garden Tuscan Bean soup; 1 small wholemeal roll or 1½ slices bread.

Evening Meals Quick

- 1 portion Chicken Tikka Masala (see recipe page 152) with herb salad.
- 1 portion Beef and Beans in Beer (see recipe page 155); 175g (cooked weight) potatoes or 150g (cooked weight) pasta or boiled rice; selection of leafy green vegetables or broccoli or cauliflower.
- 4 cod fillet fish fingers, grilled or baked; 225g mashed potato; 4 tablespoons peas; 1 portion fruit.

Evening Meals Not quite so quick

- 1 portion Tuna Lasagne (see recipe page 157); broccoli or mixed salad.
- 1 portion Catalan Egg Supper (see recipe page 159); 65g wholemeal bread.

Snacks/Treats

- 1 medium glass wine or 275ml bottle cider or lager.
- 1 Lo Bar.
- 1 slice bread with Marmite.
- 1 portion fruit with 4 pieces ready-to-eat dried apricot or prune.

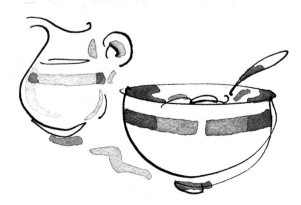

WEEK TWO

Notes

- You can choose meals from other weeks if you like, as long as you swap from the same category – e.g. Lunches for Lunches.

Breakfasts

- 1 medium bowlful porridge made with water; 40ml skimmed milk to cover plus one teaspoonful runny honey; 1 slice toast.
- 1 Müller Light yogurt; 1 apple; 1 large banana.
- 30g Fruit'n Fibre; 125ml skimmed milk; 1 slice toast and Marmite.

Lunches

- 1 pack Boots Shapers Garlic Pâté; 4 dark rye Ryvitas; salad; 1 × 125g pot French style set fruit yogurt.
- 1 can Weight Watchers soup of choice; 1 wholemeal pitta filled with 30g crumbled feta cheese, 4 stoned olives, chopped crunchy salad items, 1 dessertspoon Free Choice mayonnaise and shredded lettuce.
- 1 Boots Shapers Tuna and Pasta Salad; 1 Shapers Strawberry Sundae; 1 portion fruit.
- 1 medium poached egg; 2 slices extra-lean back bacon, grilled; 2 tomatoes, halved and grilled; 1 slice bread.
- 1 × 425g can Baxters Garden Pea soup; 1 wholemeal bap; 1 Shape fruit fromage frais.

Evening Meals Quick

- 1 portion Tangy Cheese and Potato Grill (see recipe page 158); green salad.
- 2-egg omelette cooked in non-stick pan sprayed with Fry Light, filled with mushrooms or grilled red peppers; 100g McCain oven chips or 75g piece bread; peas or salad.
- 2 large low-fat sausages, grilled; 225g mashed potato; 5 tablespoons baked beans; 1 orange.

Evening Meals Not quite so quick

- 1 portion Easy Seafood Pie (see recipe page 159); 1 portion green beans.
- 125g roast chicken (skin removed); 2 chunks average size roast potato; 1 tablespoon stuffing; 1 portion leafy greens, 1 portion carrots; gravy skimmed of fat.
- 1 portion Chilli Beef Pizza (see recipe page 155); salad.

Snacks/Treats

- 1 medium glass wine or 275ml cider or lager.
- 1 Boots Shapers Cappuccino bar.
- 2 dark rye Ryvitas, 1 level dessertspoon peanut butter.
- 15g sunflower seeds.

WEEK **THREE**

Notes

- Eat as much as you can of your unlimited salads and vegetables – they contain vitamins and minerals and will help to fill you up.

Breakfasts

- 1 Shape Twinpot bio yogurt; 1 slice toast with 2 teaspoons low-sugar jam or marmalade; 1 small fruit.
- 40g muesli with 125ml skimmed milk; ½ pink grapefruit.
- 1 English muffin with low-fat spread and 2 teaspoons low-sugar jam or marmalade; 1 portion fruit.

Lunches

- 1 St Michael 95 per cent fat-free Stonebaked Vegetable Pizza; salad.
- 1 sachet 10-calorie soup; 1 medium portion cooked chicken (skin removed); 1 small wholemeal roll with low-fat spread; salad.
- 1 McDonald's hamburger (no cheese); 1 McDonald's pure fruit juice.
- 1 × 225g baked potato topped with 1 portion Tuna Pâté (see recipe page 60); salad.
- 175g leftover cooked rice mixed with 50g chopped chicken or ham, 4 chopped dried ready-to-eat apricots, 1 dessertspoon pine nuts or sunflower seeds, chopped crisp salad vegetables, plus oil-free French dressing; 1 portion fruit.

Evening Meals Quick

- 1 portion Cheesy Gammon Pasta (see recipe page 156); salad
- 1 portion Chinese Duck with Noodles (see recipe page 153); 1 portion fruit.
- 2 Birds Eye Salmon Fish Cakes; peas; carrots; 1 pot Cadbury's Light Chocolate Mousse (or any mousse 100 calories or less) or 1 large banana.

Evening Meals Not quite so quick

- 1 portion Aubergine and Lentil Curry (see recipe page 111); 4 tablespoons (cooked weight) boiled rice.
- 1 portion Cobbler Topped Goulash (see recipe page 113); 125g potatoes; leafy greens.
- 1 portion Chilli Con Carne (see recipe page 154) with 1 portion Spicy Potato Wedges (see recipe page 158) or with 200g (cooked weight) boiled rice; salad.

Snacks/Treats

- 1 medium glass wine or 275ml cider or lager.
- 1 Boots Shapers Turkish Delight bar.
- 25g half-fat Cheddar cheese with 2 pieces Melba toast; pickled onions.
- 1 medium slice malt loaf with a little low-fat spread.

WEEK **FOUR**

Notes

- Don't forget to vary your choices as much as possible and eat plenty of fruit.

Breakfasts

- ½ can of wholewheat spaghetti in tomato sauce on 1 slice toast; 1 portion fruit.
- Medium bowlful cornflakes or branflakes with 125ml skimmed milk; 1 slice toast.
- 1 Müller Fruit Corner yogurt; 1 portion fruit.

Lunches

- 1 × 205g can Heinz Curried Beans with Sultanas on 1 slice toast; 1 Shape fruit fromage frais.
- Sandwich of 2 slices bread filled with 40g half-fat Cheddar cheese and tomato; 1 Prewetts apple and date bar.
- 1 Boots Shapers Lunchtime Selection; 1 portion fruit.
- 2 medium poached eggs, on 1½ slices toast; 1 portion fruit.
- 1 whole carton New Covent Garden Lentil and Tomato soup; 1 slice bread.

Evening Meals Quick

- 1 portion Tuna Kedgeree (see recipe page 158); green salad.
- One Quarterpounder Vegeburger, grilled or dry fried; 110g oven chips or 1 pack McCain Micro Chips; peas; 1 portion fruit.
- 1 × 110g lean gammon steak or beefsteak; 200g new potatoes; 4 tablespoons sweetcorn or broad beans; 2 rings pineapple or other fruit of choice.

Evening Meals Not quite so quick

- 125g roast leg of lamb or pork; 2 chunks roast potato; 1 spoonful mint or apple sauce; 2 portions green vegetables; thin gravy, fat skimmed.
- 1 portion Turkey and Mushroom Filo Pie (see recipe page 153); 225g new potatoes; 1 portion broccoli.

Snacks/Treats

- 1 medium glass wine or 275ml cider or lager.
- 1 Honey Malt Halo bar.
- 1 can Weight Watchers Minestrone soup, 1 Sunblest crisproll.
- 1 large banana.

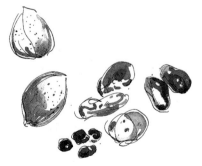

WEEK **FIVE**

Notes

- Try not to weigh yourself too often – weight fluctuates naturally a little from day to day, and even from week to week. Get a tape measure and measure your inch loss too.

Breakfasts

- 1 medium boiled or poached egg; 1 slice bread; 200ml orange juice.
- Small bowlful Fruit'n Fibre or branflakes with 125ml low-fat natural yogurt, 25ml orange juice poured over, 1 chopped apple and 1 teaspoon sesame seeds.
- 2 Weetabix with 125ml skimmed milk; 1 small banana.

Lunches

- 1 portion Tuna Pâté (see recipe page 60); 1 wholemeal bap; salad.
- 1 Findus Ham and Pineapple French Bread Pizza; 1 portion fruit; 1 Shape fruit fromage frais.
- 1 Boots Shapers triple sandwich pack; 1 portion fruit.
- 1 St Michael Layered Salad with Salmon; 1 portion fruit.
- 1 portion Spicy Potato Wedges (see recipe page 158); ¼ pack Primula Nacho dip; salad.

Evening Meals Quick

- 1 portion Chicken Satay (see recipe page 152); green salad.
- 1 piece frozen fish fillet in breadcrumbs, baked or grilled; 110g oven chips or 1 pack McCain Micro Chips or 225g mashed potatoes; peas.
- 2 medium eggs, scrambled with skimmed milk and seasoning; 2 slices extra-lean back bacon, grilled; 50g piece bread with low-fat spread.

Evening Meals Not quite so quick

- 1 portion Lamb Moussaka (see recipe page 153); mixed salad.
- 1 portion Jambalaya (see recipe page 157); mixed salad.

Snacks/Treats

- 1 medium glass wine or 275ml cider or lager.
- 2 Jaffa cakes.
- 1 bag Weight Watchers Weavers crisps.
- 25g All-Bran with 30ml skimmed milk.

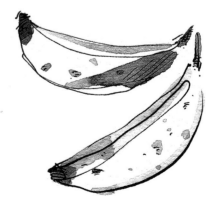

WEEK SIX

Notes

- When you have finished Week 6, turn to Chapter 10 for what to do next.

Breakfasts

- 6 tablespoons baked beans in tomato sauce on 1 slice toast; 1 portion fruit.
- 1 Müller Light yogurt; 1 large banana; 4 pieces ready-to-eat dried apricots or prunes.
- 2 slices toast; 2 teaspoons low-sugar jam or marmalade; 1 Shape fruit yogurt.

Lunches

- 50g hummus; 1 wholewheat pitta bread; chopped crisp salad items; green salad; 4 black olives.
- 1 × 405g can Heinz Lentil and Vegetable soup; 1 wholemeal bap; 1 portion fruit.
- 1 Weight Watchers Vegetable Balti with Naan bread; 1 Shape fromage frais.
- 1 portion Cauliflower Cheese with Ham (see recipe page 156); salad.
- 50g (dry weight) couscous, reconstituted and mixed with 50g cooked chopped ham or turkey, salad items, 4 pieces ready-to-eat dried apricot, chopped, and oil-free French dressing.

Evening Meals   Quick

- 1 portion Salmon Fishcakes (see recipe page 156); peas, broccoli or salad; 1 St Ivel Shape Mousse.
- 1 medium chicken breast, grilled or baked and skin removed; 225g new potatoes; 4 tablespoons sweetcorn or peas; 1 large banana.
- 1 × 225g baked potato; 1/2 400g can baked beans; 50g half-fat Cheddar, grated; salad.

Evening Meals   Not quite so quick

- 1 portion Chicken and Ham Potato Pie (see recipe page 152); carrots, greens.
- 1 portion Tagliatelle with Meatballs in Tomato Sauce (see recipe page 154); green salad.

Snacks/Treats

- 1 medium glass wine or 275ml cider or lager.
- 1 pack Weight Watchers Cookies, chocolate chip variety.
- 1 × 25g bag Go Ahead Ripplechips.
- 1 Quaker Harvest Apple and Raisin Chewy bar.

TOP 20 FAMILY RECIPES

CHICKEN TIKKA MASALA

Serves 4
475 calories and 14g fat per portion

1 dessertspoon groundnut or sunflower oil

4 boneless chicken breasts, skin removed and each cut
   into 5 or 6 slices

2 tablespoons tikka powder (not paste)

200ml full-fat Greek yogurt

Juice of a lime

Salt and pepper

200g (dry weight) basmati rice

4 dessertspoons mango chutney, to serve

Heat the oil in a non-stick lidded frying pan and stir-
fry the chicken pieces until they are beginning to turn
golden. Lower the heat and add the tikka powder,
stirring well for a minute. Add the yogurt and stir
again, then put the lid on the pan and simmer for
10 minutes, stirring once or twice. Add the lime juice
and some seasoning.

Meanwhile, cook the rice in boiling salted water
until tender (see below) and serve with the chicken
and a green leaf, coriander leaf and cucumber salad.

NOTE *I prefer the absorption method to cook rice, especially
basmati. For every 100g (dry weight) rice, add 150ml water to
the saucepan, stir well, cover with a tight-fitting lid and allow to
simmer gently for approximately 20 minutes. Check once or
twice during cooking that the rice hasn't dried out — if so, pour
a little more water in; it will quickly come back to simmer.
When the rice is cooked, all the water should be absorbed and
there is no need to drain. Simply riffle through with a fork and
serve from the saucepan.*

CHICKEN SATAY

Serves 4
500 calories and 15g fat per portion

100ml 8 per cent fat fromage frais

3 tablespoons smooth peanut butter

Juice of a lime

½ teaspoon ground cumin seed

4 boneless chicken breasts, skin removed and cut into
   bite-sized chunks

200g (dry weight) Thai fragrant rice (or white or
   wholegrain basmati rice)

5 pieces ready-to-eat dried apricot, chopped

3cm piece cucumber, chopped

In a bowl, mix together the fromage frais and peanut
butter with the lime juice and cumin seed, then add
the chicken cubes and coat well. If possible, leave to
marinate for 15 minutes.

Meanwhile, cook the rice in boiling salted water (see
Note, left). When the rice is half cooked, after about 10
minutes, thread the chicken pieces on to four skewers
and grill under a medium heat, turning occasionally.

When the rice and chicken are cooked, stir the
apricot and cucumber into the rice and serve with an
iceberg lettuce and spring onion salad.

CHICKEN AND HAM POTATO PIE

Serves 4
455 calories and 13g fat per portion

800g old potatoes

30g low-fat spread

75ml skimmed milk

Salt and black pepper

400g boneless lean chicken, cut into bite-sized pieces

100g extra-lean ham, sliced

1 tablespoon finely chopped parsley or tarragon

1 × 450g jar Homepride Low in Fat Creamy Mushroom
and Garlic Sauce

60g frozen peas, thawed

2 tablespoons ready-made golden breadcrumbs

Peel, dice and boil the potatoes in lightly salted water until tender, drain and mash with the spread and milk and a little seasoning. Set aside. In a suitably sized pie dish, mix together the chicken, ham, herbs, sauce and peas and smooth out. Top with the mashed potato and finish with the crumbs. Bake for 20–25 minutes at 180°C/350°F/Gas 4 or until the chicken is cooked. Serve with carrots and a green vegetable.

TURKEY AND MUSHROOM FILO PIE

Serves 4
340 calories and 11g fat per portion

400g turkey fillet, cut into bite-sized slices

100g extra lean ham, cut into bite-sized slices

100g small mushrooms, halved

100g frozen sweetcorn kernels, thawed

1 × 450g jar Homepride Low in Fat Creamy Stroganoff
Sauce

100g filo pastry

20ml olive oil

Place the turkey, ham, mushrooms and sweetcorn in a four-portion square pie dish and mix well. Pour over the sauce. Cut each oblong filo sheet into two, brush with a little of the oil and place over the pie, pleating it slightly, and making sure the pie is completely covered. Press down the edges and bake at 180°C/350°F/Gas 4 for 25 minutes or until golden, by which time the turkey should be cooked through. Serve with new potatoes and broccoli or green beans.

CHINESE DUCK WITH NOODLES

Serves 4
460 calories and 11g fat per portion

200g (dry weight) medium egg thread noodles

1 tablespoon groundnut or corn oil

4 duck breast fillets (about 150g each), skin removed
and thinly sliced

1 large red pepper, deseeded and thinly sliced

175g baby sweetcorn

100g mangetout

8 medium spring onions, sliced lengthways

200g fresh beansprouts

2 tablespoons light soy sauce

100ml orange juice

1 tablespoon red wine vinegar

1 tablespoon runny honey

1 dessertspoon cornflour

Soak the noodles in boiling water or according to pack instructions.

Meanwhile, heat the oil in a large non-stick frying pan or wok and stir-fry the duck, peppers, sweetcorn and mangetout for two minutes over a high heat. Add the spring onions and beansprouts and stir for a minute. Beat together the remaining ingredients and pour into the pan, stir for a minute to thicken, and serve immediately on top of the drained noodles.

LAMB MOUSSAKA

Serves 4
440 calories and 23g fat per portion

2 medium aubergines

2 tablespoons olive oil

2 medium onions, finely chopped

1 clove garlic, finely chopped

450g lean lamb fillet, minced

I dessertspoon fresh chopped oregano (or I teaspoon dried)

Salt and black pepper

I level tablespoon sun-dried tomato paste

175ml lamb stock from cube

I medium egg

I × 525g carton Napolina Creamy Pasta Lasagne Bake

2 tablespoons stale breadcrumbs

2 tablespoons grated Parmesan cheese

Top and tail the aubergines and slice into rounds about Icm thick. Place on a baking tray, brush with some of the oil and grill or bake until golden.

Heat the rest of the oil in a large non-stick frying pan and sauté the onions and garlic until soft and transparent. Add the lamb and stir to brown. Add the oregano and seasoning, sun-dried tomato paste and stock and stir well. Bring to a simmer and cook for 30 minutes, uncovered.

Spoon the mixture into a baking dish and cover with the aubergine slices. In a mixing bowl, beat the egg into the lasagne sauce and pour evenly over the aubergines. Mix the breadcrumbs with the cheese and sprinkle on top, then bake at 190°C/375°F/Gas 5 for 30 minutes or until the top is golden. Serve with a large mixed salad and oil-free dressing.

TAGLIATELLE WITH MEATBALLS IN TOMATO SAUCE

Serves 4
475 calories and 9g fat per portion

50g white bread, crusts removed and crumbed

75ml skimmed milk

350g extra-lean minced beef

I level teaspoon dried oregano

I clove garlic, crushed

Salt and black pepper

I large egg, beaten

Fry Light cooking spray

I quantity Tomato Sauce (see recipe page 107)

300g (dry weight) tagliatelle

2 tablespoons grated Parmesan cheese

Put the breadcrumbs in a bowl, pour over the milk and stir. Add the beef, oregano, garlic, salt and pepper, and combine the mixture well. Add the egg and combine again, then take I tablespoon of mixture at a time and roll into a small ball. The mixture should make around 16 balls.

Spray a non-stick frying pan with Fry Light and dry-fry the balls, turning frequently, over a medium heat, until browned. Pour the tomato sauce into the pan, bring to a simmer and cook, covered, for 15 minutes, adding a little water if the sauce dries out.

Meanwhile, cook the pasta in plenty of boiling salted water, drain and serve with the meatballs in sauce, and the Parmesan cheese sprinkled over the top. Serve with plenty of green salad.

CHILLI CON CARNE

Serves 4
300 calories and 11g fat per portion

I tablespoon corn oil

2 medium red onions, finely chopped

I stick celery, finely chopped

I large green pepper, deseeded and chopped

325g extra-lean minced beef

100ml beef stock

I × 400g can chopped tomatoes with chilli

2 tablespoons tomato purée

I dash Worcestershire sauce

I large fresh green chilli, deseeded and chopped
   (or I teaspoon chilli powder or to taste)

1 x 400g can mixed pulses, drained and well rinsed

Salt and black pepper

Chopped parsley or coriander leaf to garnish

Heat the oil in a large non-stick lidded frying pan and stir-fry the onions, celery and pepper over a medium high heat until soft. Add the beef and sauté over a medium heat, stirring a few times, until browned. Add the rest of the ingredients and stir, bring to a simmer, cover and cook for 30 minutes. Garnish with chopped parsley or coriander and serve with Spicy Potato Wedges (see recipe page 158) or with 50g (dry weight) plain boiled rice per person, and a green salad.

BEEF AND BEANS IN BEER

Serves 4
355 calories and 12g fat per portion

1 tablespoon olive oil

400g extra-lean braising steak, cubed

2 large onions, cut into wedges

2 cloves garlic, crushed

2 sticks celery, chopped

2 large carrots, peeled and sliced

1 dessertspoon fresh chopped thyme or 1 teaspoon dried

2 level tablespoons tomato purée

1 bottle (400ml) stout

200g cooked weight cannellini beans

200g mushrooms, sliced

1 dessertspoon cornflour mixed with a little water

Salt and black pepper

Heat the oil in a flameproof casserole and brown the meat. Remove the meat with a slotted spoon and reserve, then add the onions to the pan and sauté for a few minutes. Add the garlic, celery and carrots and stir for another minute. Return the meat to the pan with

the thyme, tomato purée and stout, bring to a simmer and cook in a preheated oven at 170°C/325°F/Gas 3 for an hour. Add the beans and mushrooms to the casserole, stir and cook for a further 30 minutes. Stir the cornflour mixture into the pan and cook for another 10 minutes. Season, then serve with 175g potatoes, or 150g (cooked weight) rice or pasta, and a green vegetable.

CHILLI BEEF PIZZA

Serves 4
424 calories and 14g fat per portion

225g extra-lean minced beef

50ml beef stock

1 fresh red chilli, deseeded and chopped

1 x 235g jar Old El Paso Taco Sauce, hot or mild

4 spring onions, thinly sliced

2 x 200g deep crust Giovanni's pizza bases
    from two pack*

2 tomatoes, sliced

75g half-fat grated mozzarella

1 small green pepper, deseeded and chopped

Put the minced beef in a non-stick frying pan and heat it up over a gentle heat until the fat starts to run, then increase the heat and cook, stirring from time to time, until well browned. Pour off any surplus fat. Add the stock, chilli, sauce and onions to the pan and cook for 20 minutes, stirring occasionally, until you have a rich sauce. (If the mixture gets too dry, add a little water.) Leave to cool a little. Heat the oven to 200°C/400°F/Gas 6, then spread the sauce over the pizza bases, and finish with slices of tomato, some green pepper and the grated mozzarella. Bake for 15 minutes or until the cheese is melted and the pizza is golden round the edges. Serve with a large mixed salad.

* IF YOU GET NAPOLINA DEEP CRUST BASES ADD 90 CALORIES PER PORTION.

CAULIFLOWER CHEESE WITH HAM

Serves 4
320 calories and 10g fat per portion

2 medium cauliflowers, broken into florets

350g extra-lean ham, cut into strips

25g low-fat spread

1 tablespoon plain flour

400ml skimmed milk, warmed

75g mature half-fat Cheddar, grated

Salt and black pepper

1 level teaspoon mustard powder

2 good-sized tomatoes, sliced thinly

2 tablespoons grated Parmesan cheese (preferably fresh)

2 tablespoons Red Leicester cheese

Boil the cauliflower florets in a little salted water until just tender.

Meanwhile, make a cheese sauce. In a small non-stick saucepan, melt the low-fat spread and add the flour, stirring over a low heat for a few minutes. Gradually add the warm milk, stirring, until you have a smooth sauce. Stir in the half-fat Cheddar, the seasoning and mustard.

Drain the cauliflower and place it in a four-serving shallow baking dish (small lasagne dish or similar). Arrange the ham around the cauliflower. Pour the sauce over the cauliflower evenly, arrange tomato slices all around the edge of the dish and sprinkle with the two cheeses. Bake or grill until the top is golden. Serve with salad and 65g crusty bread per portion.

CHEESY GAMMON PASTA

Serves 4
490 calories and 12g fat per portion

1 x 225g lean gammon steak (without fat)

250g (dry weight) pasta shells or bows

100g Boursin Leger cheese

8 black olives, stoned and halved

16 cherry tomatoes, halved

1 jar mixed peppers in tomato sauce

100g half-fat mozzarella cheese

Fresh basil (optional)

Grill the gammon steak and cut into bite-sized pieces.

Meanwhile, boil the pasta in salted water until tender and drain, and combine in a heatproof shallow serving dish with the Boursin Leger cheese, then add the olives, tomatoes and peppers in sauce. Stir in the gammon, then thinly slice the mozzarella and arrange over the top. Pop under the grill for a couple of minutes until the mozzarella is melted. Garnish with basil leaves and serve straight away with a green salad.

SALMON FISHCAKES

Serves 4
417 calories and 16g fat per portion

800g old potatoes

25g low-fat spread

75ml skimmed milk

250g salmon fillet

1 tablespoon chopped fresh parsley

Salt and black pepper

1 level tablespoon plain flour

100g plain breadcrumbs

2 tablespoons corn or groundnut oil

Peel the potatoes and cut into chunks; boil in salted water until tender, drain and mash in a large bowl with the low-fat spread and skimmed milk.

Meanwhile, poach or microwave the salmon for a few minutes (don't overcook) and flake into the bowl with the potato. Add the parsley and seasoning and, using the flour on a board or clean work surface to coat, form into eight fishcakes. Place the breadcrumbs on a large plate and dip the cakes into this to coat each well. Heat the oil in a non-stick frying pan and fry the fishcakes, turning once, until golden. Serve immediately, with peas and broccoli.

TUNA LASAGNE

Serves 4
500 calories and 12g fat per portion

1 tablespoon olive oil

1 large leek or onion, thinly sliced

1 × 400g can chopped tomatoes with herbs

1 level tablespoon tomato purée

100ml fish stock or thereabouts

400g white fish fillet

400g canned tuna in brine or water, well drained

100g sliced mushrooms

8 lasagne sheets, no-need-to-precook variety

1 carton Napolina Creamy Pasta Bake for Tuna

75g half-fat mozzarella, grated

Heat the oil in a large non-stick frying pan and sauté the leek or onion until soft and transparent. Add the tomatoes, tomato purée and fish stock, stir and simmer for a few minutes. Cut the fish fillet into bite-sized pieces and add to the pan; flake the tuna and add with the mushrooms. Bring to a simmer and remove from heat.

Spoon half the tuna mixture evenly into the base of a four-serving lasagne dish and arrange half the lasagne sheets over. Spoon the rest of the tuna over, arrange the last four lasagne sheets on top, then pour over the sauce. Sprinkle the grated mozzarella on top and bake at 190°C/375°F/Gas 5 for 25 minutes or until bubbling and golden. Serve with broccoli or a green salad.

NOTE *Don't worry if the tomato and fish sauce seems rather runny when you spoon it into the dish. The no-precook lasagne absorbs liquid when it bakes and the resulting dish will not be too moist at all. Without this extra liquid the lasagne sheets will not cook properly.*

JAMBALAYA

Serves 4
490 calories and 12g fat per portion

2 tablespoons corn or sunflower oil

225g diced chicken meat (skin removed)

1 large onion, finely chopped

1 yellow pepper and 1 red pepper, deseeded and chopped

2 cloves garlic, crushed

1 large red fresh chilli, deseeded and chopped

300g (dry weight) long-grain rice

900ml chicken or vegetable stock

1 average chorizo sausage, sliced into thin rounds

100g chopped tomatoes

225g peeled prawns

Heat the oil in a large non-stick frying pan and brown the chicken pieces; remove with a slotted spoon and reserve. Sauté the onion in the pan until soft and just turning golden, adding the pepper and garlic halfway through. Add the chilli and stir again, then add the rice, stock, chorizo and tomatoes, stir, cover, and simmer for 20 minutes or until the rice has absorbed all the liquid. Stir in the prawns a minute or two before serving with a salad.

TUNA KEDGEREE

Serves 4
460 calories and 14g fat per portion

1 tablespoon corn oil

1 medium onion, finely chopped

1 clove garlic, crushed

1 dessertspoon mild curry powder

225g basmati rice

750ml fish stock

450g fresh or frozen tuna, defrosted and cut into chunks

100g petit pois, thawed

Salt and black pepper

3 medium eggs, hard-boiled

Fresh parsley, chopped, to garnish

Heat the oil in a non-stick frying pan and sauté the onion until soft and transparent. Add the garlic and curry powder and stir for a minute more, then add the rice and stock and stir well. Bring to a simmer, cover and cook gently for 20 minutes. Add the tuna and peas and simmer for a further 5 minutes, adding a little more fish stock if necessary. Season to taste. Check that the rice is tender. Cut the eggs into quarters, then into eighths. When the tuna rice is cooked, sprinkle the eggs on top and serve garnished.

SPICY POTATO WEDGES

Serves 4
215 calories and 5g fat per portion

4 x 250g baking potatoes, cleaned

1 tablespoon olive oil

1 pack Schwartz Tomato and Herb coating

$\frac{1}{2}$ teaspoon ground paprika

Slice the potatoes into four lengthways, then again into eight wedges. Place on a baking sheet and brush the oil over. Sprinkle on the tomato and herb coating and the paprika. Bake at 200°C/400°F/Gas 6 for 40 minutes or until cooked through, crisp and golden. Serve immediately with Chilli con Carne (see recipe page 154), or with a low-fat ready-made dip or a mix of Greek yogurt, chopped cucumber and garlic.

TANGY CHEESE AND POTATO GRILL

Serves 4
425 calories and 13.5g fat per portion

900g old potatoes

8 extra-lean bacon rashers

Black pepper

1 whole quantity tomato sauce (see recipe page 107)

100g half-fat mozzarella, grated

4 tablespoons grated Parmesan (preferably fresh)

1 tablespoon chopped fresh basil, to garnish

Peel the potatoes, cut into large chunks and boil in salted water for 15 minutes or until just cooked but not breaking up. Cut into thick slices.

Meanwhile, cut the bacon rashers into 2 or 3 pieces each and dry-fry in a non-stick pan. Place the potatoes evenly in the base of a shallow heatproof serving dish and arrange the bacon around the potatoes. Season with pepper. Pour the tomato sauce over, coating everything well, and top with the grated cheeses. Grill for a few minutes until the cheese is bubbling. Garnish and serve with green salad.

EASY SEAFOOD PIE

Serves 4
482 calories and 11g fat per portion

600g white fish fillet

550ml skimmed milk

1 bay leaf

Salt and white pepper

2 medium eggs, hard-boiled

50g small mushrooms, sliced

100g frozen peas, cooked and drained

30g low-fat spread

1 tablespoon plain flour

1 tablespoon chopped parsley

Juice of ¼ lemon

1 × 280g pack frozen or chilled seafood cocktail, thawed

800g (cooked weight) instant mashed potato

50g half-fat Cheddar cheese, grated

Put the fish fillet in a frying pan with the milk, bay leaf and seasoning and simmer for 10 minutes or until lightly cooked. Drain off the milk from the pan and reserve. Flake the fish lightly and arrange in the base of a four-serving pie dish. Chop the eggs and arrange them with the mushrooms and peas around the fish. Heat the fat in a non-stick saucepan over a medium heat, add the flour and stir for a minute. Slowly add the reserved milk, stirring, until you have a smooth sauce. Check the seasoning and add the parsley and lemon.

Arrange the seafood cocktail in the pie dish, pour over the sauce and top with the mashed potato and grated Cheddar. Bake at 190°C/375°F/Gas 5 for 25 minutes or until golden. Serve with green beans.

CATALAN EGG SUPPER

Serves 4
365 calories and 11.5g fat per portion

400g new potatoes, cleaned

1 large onion, thinly sliced

1 tablespoon olive oil

2 red peppers, deseeded and sliced

Salt and black pepper

1 × 400g can chopped tomatoes with herbs

100g frozen sweetcorn, thawed

400g canned tuna in brine or water, drained

4 large eggs

Cut the potatoes into bite-sized chunks and boil in salted water until cooked; drain and reserve.

Meanwhile, heat the oil in a large non-stick lidded frying pan and sauté the onion until turning soft. Add the red peppers and stir for a few minutes to soften. Season, add the chopped tomatoes and bring to a simmer and cook gently for 10 minutes. Add the potatoes and sweetcorn, stir, then cook again for 10 minutes. Remove from the heat, gently stir in the tuna, then spoon the mixture into one large or four individual gratin dish/es. Make four wells in the mixture and break an egg into each well; season and bake in the oven for 15 minutes at 180°C/350°F/Gas 4 until the eggs are just set but the yolks still runny. Serve immediately with a green salad and 65g wholemeal bread, which will add 140 calories to the meal.

CASE HISTORY

ESTHER AND GUY DICKENS

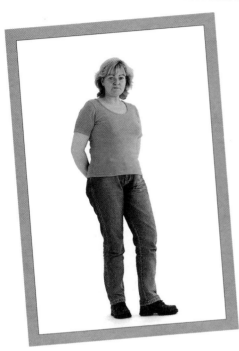

ESTHER DICKENS

AGE: **38**

STATUS: **Married to Guy; one 15-year-old son**

OCCUPATION: **Housewife**

HEIGHT: **5 ft 4 ins**

STARTING WEIGHT: **11 st 12 lb**

WEIGHT AFTER SIX WEEKS: **10 st 10 lb**

STARTING BMI: **29.5**

BMI after six weeks: **26.6**

STARTING STATISTICS: **40½–34½–44**

STATISTICS AFTER SIX WEEKS: **38½–33–41**

When Esther and her husband Guy sent me their food diary, I could see straight away why they were both quite a lot overweight. They had been eating a diet extremely high in fat, sometimes eating red meat three times a day, plus snacks like full-fat cheese and eggs.

It was nothing out of the ordinary for them to have a cooked breakfast with bacon or sausage, spaghetti Bolognese or egg and chips for lunch, a beef stew at teatime, and then cheese for a late supper. I estimated that their daily fat intake was at least 45 per cent of their total daily calories, rather than the 30 per cent or so it should have been. And their total daily calorie intake was about 25 per cent more than necessary for an average adult. As both Esther and Guy are slightly shorter than average they were eating far too much – to put it bluntly!

As Guy is at home a lot and Esther's son Lee eats with them, I put them on the Family Plan – but I admit that I had my doubts about whether they'd stick with it!

I needn't have worried. Both Esther and Guy threw themselves into their vastly changed diet with enthusiasm, and embraced the concept of exercise with equal gusto.

Says Esther, 'Even if you hadn't taken us on, we decided we were going to get slimmer and fitter, and eat more healthily. I had had a weight problem almost all my life. I tend to eat when I'm sad, for comfort, which is a hard habit to break but with your help and doing it together with Guy, I felt I could do it.

'I hated my bum and "saddle bags" and wanted to look better, but also I would like to have another baby and feel that I must be in good shape before conceiving, so that was a strong motivation.

'The six-week programme has been very good for me – I found the food great, there was lots of choice, and I can't honestly say I felt hungry. I love being able to eat things like tortillas, ice cream and so on. The menus were fabulous! My hardest time for some reason was on the sixth day when I felt like chips – but had new potatoes instead (though we do still eat small portions of chips sometimes). My son Lee enjoyed the meals too; he is tall and thin but found them satisfying if he had extra potatoes and so on.

'We realise now just how much fat and food we were eating before – but at the time we didn't. Now we know how to cut back on fat and know what we **CAN** eat, I'm sure we'll stick with this way of eating.'

Because Esther and Guy are young, took a lot of exercise during the six weeks, and their previous diet when they began the Family Plan had been so high in calories and fat, the weight came off them easily. Both Esther and Guy actually lost a little over the stone in the six weeks but I wasn't worried because I knew they were both eating plenty and looked and felt so fit and well.

Even when the family went on holiday to Ibiza, they managed to lose weight. 'We did have more treats that week but we swam all the time and danced all night, so we burnt off more calories!' said Esther.

'For exercise, my preference was walking, which I shall definitely keep up. I have more energy, feel stronger, and people have made comments on my hair, skin, eyes and posture being better, so my confidence in myself has improved. Guy says I look sexier and my love life has improved because I'm not so ashamed of my body.'

Esther would like to reach 10 stone or a bit less, which will bring her BMI down to just under 25, which she should not find a problem to maintain as she feels that now her life is looking so good and she has a goal to aim for (another child!) comfort eating won't pose a problem.

Debenhams' Casual Club T-shirt, Jasper Conran jeans and Trader velvet trimmed cardigan. Grattan ankle boots

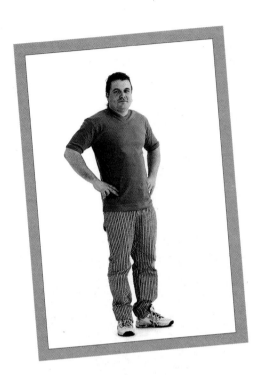

GUY DICKENS

AGE: **27**
STATUS: **Married to Esther**
OCCUPATION: **Self-employed in transport**
HEIGHT: **5 ft 6 ins**
STARTING WEIGHT: **12 st 11 lb**
WEIGHT AFTER SIX WEEKS: **11 st 8 lb**
STARTING BMI: **29.9**
BMI AFTER SIX WEEKS: **27**
STARTING STATISTICS: **Chest – 41**
   Waist – 37
STATISTICS AFTER SIX WEEKS: **Chest – 39½**
   Waist – 33½

Though Guy wasn't a fat child, by the age of 16 he weighed 12 stone, and at 23 was 14½ stone. 'I never thought about weight because I wasn't worried about it at the time, but thinking back, all the food I ate was fried.' Despite managing to lose three stone then on a crash diet, most of it came back on and Guy had been stuck at around 13 stone for some time. He now realises, along with Esther, that he made the mistake of returning to most of his old eating habits, eating far too much fat, and also drinking too much beer.

'I hate the way my face looked before the plan – I put weight on my face more than anywhere else!' For health reasons, too, Guy wanted to lose weight although he didn't want to lose too much as he 'pumps iron' in the gym regularly and can benchpress 80kgs.

'Beer is still a weakness, but not as much as it was, because I am more motivated. I found almost everything about the plan surprising – how it never felt like a strict diet; in fact I never felt like I was dieting. A few times I had more beer than I was supposed to but it didn't affect the result – and my tastebuds just don't find rich fatty foods that appealing any more.

'Ideally I would like to lose just a few more pounds and then maintain it with regular exercise. I think you can eat everything in moderation – that's the key.'

Says Esther, 'I think he looks great – he looks so much younger now, yet before we started slimming he was worried that he was soon going to look older than his dad.'

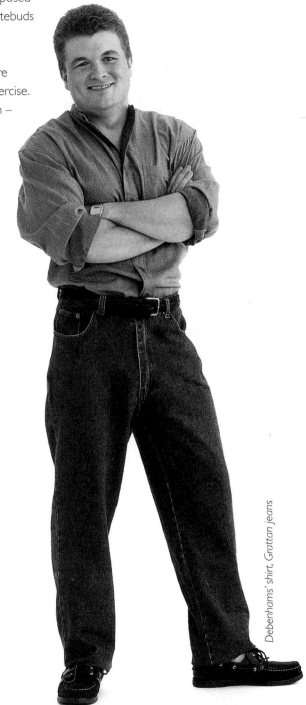

Debenhams' shirt, Grattan jeans

the 'e' word

Tone Up and Burn Up – On Your Own Terms

E is for Exercise – which most of us seem to hate.

E is for Exercise – for which most of us can't find time.

And E is for Exercise – which is the single most important thing a person can do for his or her well-being and confidence, now and through life.

This, then, is the dilemma. This chapter sets out to increase your motivation to exercise, and to show you how to do it with minimum misery and disruption to your busy schedule.

Short-term Motivating Factors

Exercise helps you lose weight! The fact is, without regular activity in the short term, you are unlikely to lose that stone in the six weeks. Exercise burns up calories and the six-week plan incorporates the idea of ½ lb a week burnt through extra exercise. In other words, if you are going to lose a stone, 3 lb of that will be weight lost through activity rather than just eating less.

In the short term, also, you will want to improve your figure by doing exercise to tone it up – you don't want to be left with flabby bits because you've lost the weight but didn't do a few minutes a day of toning work.

And in the short term, you will enjoy the sense of achievement and self-control that comes from beginning an activity programme and realising that your body is feeling better as well as looking better.

Long-term Motivating Factors

In the long term, exercise has so many benefits that I can hardly find room to list them all. Here are some of the main ones:

- Exercise of all kinds helps you to maintain a suitable weight for the rest of your life. All research shows that people who exercise regularly have the least problems with their weight.
- Exercise keeps your heart and lungs fit. Aerobic exercise, such as brisk walking, cycling, step class or swimming targets your heart and lungs and increases their strength and capacity.

  There is then less risk of cardiovascular problems, heart disease, stroke, heart attack and so on. There is also less chance of circulatory problems and feeling cold!

- Exercise helps to prevent osteoporosis, the decline in bone mass which affects the majority of women past menopause and some men and can lead to debility and fractures in older age.
- Exercise can improve posture and help prevent back pain and stress-related aches and pains.
- Exercise can make you stronger.
- Exercise can help to control diabetes, and can help to prevent or control arthritis.
- Exercise can improve energy levels, mood, brain power, concentration and hearing, and reduce insomnia, stress, anxiety and tension.
- Exercise can help to regulate women's periods and reduce PMT symptoms. It can also help to prevent incontinence and prolapse in later years.
- Exercise can improve the condition of skin, eyes and hair.

So you see, isn't it a pity that you don't like or find time for exercise?

Doing it on your own terms

You need to do two sorts of exercise regularly:

- Aerobic exercise to help burn calories, get your heart and lungs fit and help you to feel great.
- Strength, tone and stretch exercise in the form of a simple routine you can do on your sitting room or bedroom floor. This is to tone your body up, help it to look slimmer, improve your posture and make you stronger and more supple.

I am sure that you can fit in both types of exercise at least three times a week, not only for the next six weeks, but for the rest of your life. Below I explain the '3 lb Factor' – your main motivation to do aerobic

exercise – and I present a simple way for you to ensure that you do your ½ lb's worth of aerobic exercise every week, in a style to suit yourself.

Later in the chapter, I have enlisted the brilliant help of Sarah McClurey, one of the UK's most popular personal trainers, to help provide you with an adaptable tone, strength and stretch programme that will work for your body, within your lifestyle. Ten minutes, four or five times a week, is all it will take to get you shaped up.

All exercise really means is using your body as it was meant to be used. So turn over and let's get started.

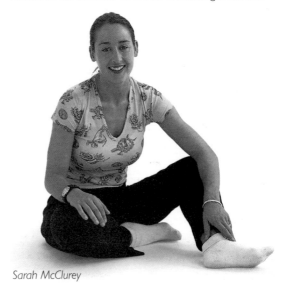

Sarah McClurey

The 3 lb Factor

You can burn up 3 lb of fat in 6 weeks.

The two main complaints people have about exercise are that it is boring, and that it doesn't slot in with their lifestyles.

Well, the '3 lb Factor' plan to help you burn off ½ pound of fat a week overcomes both those problems.

In order to burn ½ lb a week, you need to burn off about 1,750 calories over and above those you normally burn. That is an extra 250 calories a day on average.

So I have designed for you a simple chart listing calorie expenditure in 50 activities and the time it will take you to burn off 50 calories, 100 calories or 250 calories doing them.

All you have to do is mix and match your activities every day to a total of 250 and you'll burn that ½ lb of fat. The chart lists the activities in order, starting with those that burn calories quickest, and finishing with the slower ones.

You can pick things you enjoy, that you are capable of doing, and do them in your own time. For instance, to make up a day's calorie burning you could pick:

5 blocks of 50-calorie burn-ups

OR

3 blocks of 50-calorie burn-ups plus one block of 100-calorie burn-up

OR

2 blocks of 100-calorie burn-ups plus one 50-calorie block

OR

1 block of 250-calorie burn-up.

It is up to you. However, here are some notes to help you decide:

- Not all the activities listed will provide you with aerobic benefits – i.e. not all will necessarily improve your heart/lung (cardiovascular) fitness. For this you need to pick an activity that raises your heart rate to a training level and maintain it for at least 15 minutes. There is no real need to get too technical about this – you will know if you are exercising at a training level if you are slightly 'puffed' while doing the exercise – i.e. your lungs are working harder and you maybe can feel your heart beating. You shouldn't feel pain or exhaustion, but you do need to feel you are working. The items marked with a * are those that are ideal aerobic activities; and if you pick them in blocks which provide at least 15 minutes of

training, then your cardiovascular system will get fitter. (Use your common sense when choosing sports such as football, rugby, netball and basketball: if you are standing around waiting for the ball, that isn't aerobic – you need to be moving around briskly for it to count.)

For the full benefits of exercise as described earlier, it is wise to build at least three blocks of aerobic exercise into your life every week, spacing them out evenly through the week.

All the other activities still burn extra calories, either through short bursts of activity (which don't count as aerobic) or through using your muscles for strength.

- If you are very unfit, pick easy types of exercise. I would always go for walking if you are unsure of your fitness, as you can build up your fitness safely and gradually. Then when you are fitter, you can try some of the more demanding activities. If you are unfit and haven't exercised in years, I would have a medical check-up too.

Activities marked with a + are those to save for when you are fitter, or to avoid if you have any medical problems.

- When exercising, wear suitable clothing and don't do vigorous exercise without warming up gently and cooling down afterwards (for example by slowly walking round the room or marching on the spot). You can also do the stretches that accompany the 10-minute tone up (see page 169).

50 Ways to Burn Up Your Daily 250 Calories

* – aerobic + – for fitter people only

Activity	Time taken to burn		
	50 calories (in mins)	100 calories (in mins)	250 calories (in mins)
Squash*+	3½	7	17½
Running*+	4¼	8½	21½
Skipping*	4½	9	22½
Cycling, racing speed*+	4½	9	22½
Cross-country running*+	5	10	25
Stair climbing* (or stair machine)	5	10	25
Healthrider*	5½	11	27½
Swimming, crawl*+	5½	11	27½
Backpacking*+	5½	11	27½
Circuit training	6	12	30
Climbing hills*+	6	12	30
Jogging*+	6¼	12½	31½
Skiing cross-country*+	6¼	12½	31½
Hockey*+	6½	13	32½
Kickboxing+	6½	13	32½
Swimming, breast*	6½	13	32½
Walking, uphill*	6½	13	32½
Horse riding, trot	7	14	35
Netball*	7	14	35
Tennis	7	14	35
Rowing (or machine)	7	14	35
Badminton	7½	15	37½
Cycling, fast*+	7½	15	37½
Dancing, disco*	7½	15	37½
Dancing, line*	7½	15	37½
Digging, heavy	7½	15	37½
Football*+	7½	15	37½
Skiing, downhill*+	7½	15	37½
Mowing, non power-driven*	7½	15	37½
Aerobics class*	8	16	40
Rugby*+	8	16	40
Walking, brisk*	8	16	40
Basketball*	10	20	50
Golf	10	20	50
Gymnastics	10	20	50
Ice skating*	10	20	50
Fencing	10	20	50
Rollerblading*+	10	20	50
Volleyball	10	20	50
Table tennis	11	22	55
Canoeing*	12½	25	62½
Cycling, slow*	12½	25	62½
Polishing	12½	25	62½
Vacuuming	12½	25	62½
Window cleaning	12½	25	62½
Bowls	16½	33	82½
Cricket, batting	16½	33	82½
Cricket, bowling	16½	33	82½
Dancing, ballroom*	16½	33	82½
Horse riding, walk	16½	33	82½

Choose your 10-minute tone up

To get the most benefit from your six-week programme, you need to tone up your muscles as well as burn off calories. This will help you to look sleeker and slimmer and so is well worth doing.

Sarah McClurey, whose London-based Professional Fitness Management (0181-942 0289) is one of the most respected teams of personal trainers in the UK, has devised a simple mix and match programme so that you can do the exercises you need for your own body, and do them when you like.

There is a set of five **STRETCHES** which should be done at the start of any toning exercise session – they will take only 1½ minutes.

Then there is a set of four **UPPER BODY** exercises – ideal for toning and strengthening your chest or bust and for getting rid of those flabby bits at the backs of your upper arms (triceps).

There is a set of four **MID SECTION** exercises for your abdominals – the ones we all need for a firm and flat stomach and a smaller waistline.

Lastly there is a set of six **LOWER BODY** exercises which will help you firm and tone up your bottom, hips, thighs and other leg muscles.

Each of these three sections will take up to five minutes to do, depending on how many repeats you are doing. You can choose whether to do one, two, or all three (plus the stretches).

For maximum results in six weeks, Sarah recommends that you do at least two of the three sections, and do them on most days. This will take you only a little over 10 minutes. If you have time to do all three sessions then you will be getting a complete body workout in about 15 minutes. But if you want to do just one section, it will take as little as 6½ minutes. It is up to you.

Another idea is to do one section on one day, then another on the following day, so that you get through all the different sections at least twice each week. If you are unfit this may be your best solution, as the worked muscles get a chance to rest the following day. As you get stronger you can always add extra sections when you have time.

Tips

- Exercise in a warm room wearing suitable clothing on a mat, towel or carpet. Do warm-up first.
- Concentrate on doing the exercises as well as possible – focusing on the muscle/s you are working.
- Always start with a good body posture (see below): knees relaxed, tummy tucked in, bottom tucked in, shoulders relaxed and down.

- Do as many repeats as you can to the point where the working muscle is tired but not exhausted. You will soon build up strength and be able to do more.
- Don't go too fast – exercises need to be controlled.
- At the end of the session it is important that you repeat the warm-up stretches to cool down and lengthen the muscles.

Posture

A good body posture can take pounds off you instantly – so try to get in the habit of standing, walking, sitting, even lying, with your body well aligned. Correct posture is also important when doing toning exercises. So look at the 'before' and 'after' photos here and try to get your own body looking like the 'after', and make it a permanent habit.

Before

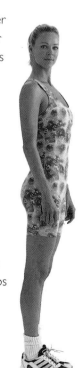

Back is in a 'letter S' with shoulder blades sticking out and the lower back forced inwards, which results in the stomach sagging out, the waist 'sinking into itself', chest disappearing, chin pointing downwards and knees locking.

After

If the spine is straightened (though not completely as you want a little natural curve in it) the bust lifts, the stomach flattens and the neck lengthens. This gives a much cleaner, slimmer look and helps prevent muscular imbalance.

STRETCHES

Shoulder Stretch

Stand with the basic correct posture with feet hip-width apart. Raise your arms above your head and stretch upwards; hold for 10–15 seconds. This also stretches the back/waist and abdominals.

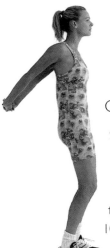

Chest Stretch

Stand as shown with knees relaxed. Clasp your hands behind your back and raise them upwards as far as you can to feel the stretch in your chest. Hold for 10–15 seconds.

Quad Stretch

Stand with correct posture, and bring right foot behind you up towards your buttocks (supporting yourself if you need to), clasping it with your right hand, keeping your knees aligned. Hold for 10–15 seconds, feeling the stretch in your right thigh. Repeat to the other side.

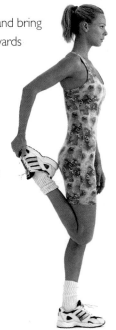

Hamstring Stretch

Keeping your back flat and abdominals pulled in, bend forward with your right leg bent and left leg straight as shown, left toes up. Place your hands on your right thigh as shown and hold for 10–15 seconds, feeling the stretch in your left hamstring (back of thigh). Repeat to other side.

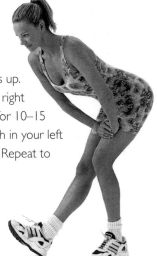

Calf Stretch

Stand with your palms flat against a wall as shown, straightening the left leg out behind you, with the right leg bent, being careful not to allow the right knee to bend beyond the toes. Both feet should be flat to the floor. Hold for 10–15 seconds, feeling a stretch down the left calf. Repeat to the other side.

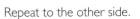

UPPER BODY SECTION

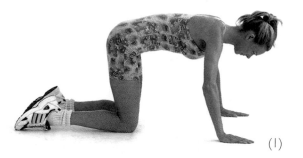

(1)

Box Press-ups

Kneel on all fours, placing your hands slightly wider apart than the width of your chest, and facing slightly

inwards. Keep pelvis tucked under and abdominals tight (1). Lower your chest to the floor, keeping shoulders in line with wrists and head in line with body. Try to aim for 10 repeats and increase when you're ready (2).

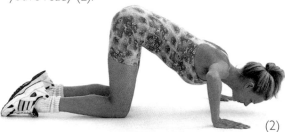

(2)

Behind Back Push

Stand in the correct position as before. Put the ball in your hands behind your back as shown and, keeping your shoulders relaxed, press/squeeze the ball. Repeat 10 times and increase when you're ready.

Ball Press

Standing with your feet hip-width apart and in correct posture, hold the ball 10 inches from your chest and push hands together, squeezing the ball. Repeat 10 times and increase repeats when you feel stronger.

Seated Triceps Dips

Sitting upright, put your hands on the floor to the sides of your hips, then move the hands back about 5 inches. Pull in the abdominals and keep back straight. Raise bottom off floor (1).

(1)

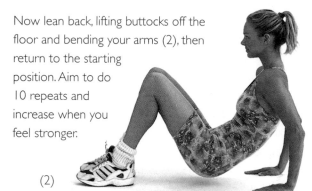

Now lean back, lifting buttocks off the floor and bending your arms (2), then return to the starting position. Aim to do 10 repeats and increase when you feel stronger.

(2)

MID SECTION

Abdominal Contractions

Lie on your back with legs bent and feet flat on floor, slightly apart. The lower back should be flat to the floor but don't press it down, as you will be flexing the spine rather than placing it in its natural position. Your legs and buttocks should be relaxed.

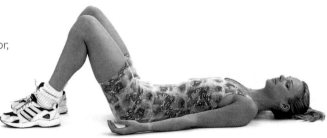

Now concentrate on pulling your abdominals in. Hold for 2–3 seconds, then relax and repeat for about a minute, breathing steadily all the time. This exercise will enable you to concentrate on your abdominals, so when you move on to the next exercise your technique will be great. This exercise can be done at any time, not necessarily lying down – walking, shopping, at your desk. The more you do it the stronger your abdominals will get.

Abdominal Curls

shoulders up from the floor. Don't pull on the head and don't lift your lower back off the floor. Imagine you have a tennis ball under your chin and that will make sure you hold your head correctly (2). Curl up (1 second), then slowly lower to floor (1 second). Start by doing 10 repeats of this exercise and build up as you feel stronger.

(1)

Start in the same body position as above, with hands lightly supporting the head to the sides or behind (1). The most important thing to remember is that the head is the heaviest part of the body and your neck will take a lot of strain if you are not supported, so find the position that feels most comfortable for you. Concentrate on your abdominals and, keeping them contracted, gently raise your head and

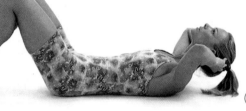

(2)

Abdominal Obliques

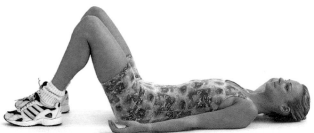

(1)

Start in the same body position as above, but this time with your right arm bent and right hand lightly on right ear, left arm at side as shown (1). Now raise your head and shoulders off the floor, keeping your abdominals contracted, but this time aim towards your left knee. Hold for 1–2 seconds, then lower and repeat to the right side. Aim to do 10 repeats (5 each side), increasing the number as you feel stronger.

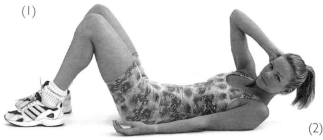

(2)

Reverse Curl

Lie on your back and raise knees in towards chest, lift legs in the air as shown, keeping knees relaxed. Place your hands on the floor beside you or across your chest and pull in the abdominal muscles (1).

Now, keeping the abdominals tight, raise your buttocks off the floor slightly (2). This need not be a big movement. Hold for a second, then lower back down to the floor. Start by doing 5 repeats of this exercise and increase them gradually as you get stronger.

(1)

(2)

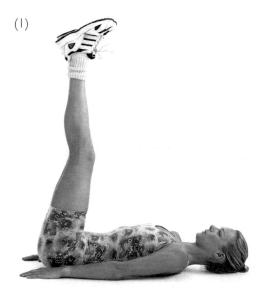

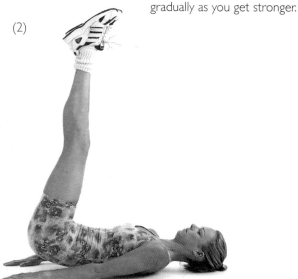

LOWER BODY SECTION

Pelvic Tilt with Crossover

This one is for the gluteals (buttocks). Lie on your back with knees bent, feet flat to the floor and hip-width apart. Now cross left leg over right as shown (1). Raise hips off floor and contract buttocks for 1–2 seconds (2),

relax and lower to floor and repeat ten times, then change legs and repeat on the other side 10 times. Increase the amount of repeats when you feel stronger.

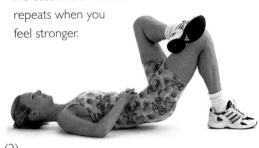

(1)

(2)

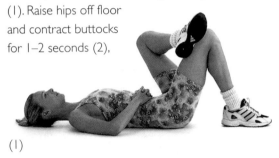

Squats

These firm up all your leg muscles. Stand with feet hip-width apart, feet facing forward. Keep your head up and abdominals in. Imagine you are slowly going to sit down on a chair. Squat down until your thighs are parallel to the floor – never let your buttocks go lower than your knees. Hold for 1–2 seconds, then come up again, contracting your buttocks as you do so. Repeat 10 times, increasing as you get stronger.

Lying Abductor

For the outer thighs and hips. Lie on your left side with left arm outstretched to support head, right hand on floor in front of you for support, abdominals contracted and left leg bent at the knee as shown (1). Lift your right leg towards the ceiling, with the knee and hip facing forwards. Don't roll your body backwards (2). Hold for 1–2 seconds and lower leg back to start. Aim to do 10 repetitions, then turn over and repeat on the other side. Increase repeats as you get stronger.

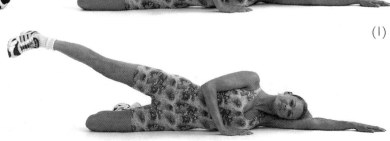

(1)

(2)

Lunges

Another one for the whole leg. Stand with feet hip-width apart, hands by your sides. Now make a big step forward with your right leg until your upper thigh is parallel with the floor, allowing your left leg to bend so that it will go down towards the floor (but don't touch the floor). Hold for 1–2 seconds, then come back to start position and repeat on the other leg. Always remember never to let your leading knee go forward over the toes, the angle should be 90 degrees. Repeat 5 times each side and build up repeats as you can.

Pliés

These work the whole leg. Stand with your feet slightly wider than hip-width apart, back straight, abdominals contracted and pelvis tucked under. Bend your knees, making sure that you don't let your buttocks go lower than knee level and that toes are in line with knees. Hold for 1–2 seconds, then slowly rise, contracting your buttocks as you do so. Aim to do 10 repeats, increasing as you feel stronger.

Inner Thigh Press

For flabby inner thighs, little works – but this does. Lie on your back with knees bent, feet flat to the floor and hip-width apart. Place a soft pliable ball between your knees (1). Now slightly raise your hips off the floor,

keeping your lower back in contact with the ground. Squeeze the ball with your knees (2), then relax a little. Repeat 10 times and increase repeats and knee pressure when you feel stronger.

Make sure you repeat the stretches for lower body as in the warm-up.

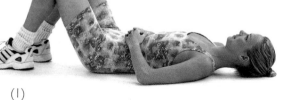

(1)

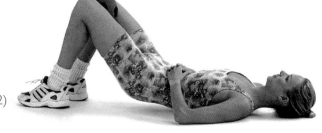

(2)

now keep that stone off for good

It isn't the slimming that is the tough thing for a lot of people, but keeping it off once it's gone! Some reports say that up to 90 per cent of people who have lost weight will, eventually, put it back on again.

This chapter is concerned with how you can avoid that risk.

The Energy Balance

There is no mystery about what will keep your weight stable once you've lost what you want to lose. It's called maintaining the 'energy balance' or taking in, in the form of calories, however many your body can use in energy expenditure – and no more.

As explained in Question 10, Chapter 2, it isn't true that ex-dieters have to eat less than non-ex-dieters in order to stay slim. Most ex-dieters should be able to eat the national average of calories (about 1,940 a day for women and 2,550 for men) and not put on weight. What you can't do is go back to eating the amount you ate when you were overweight – then the weight **WILL** come straight back on (unless you do much more exercise than you used to do then: a topic we'll deal with later). Remember – you got fat because you were eating more than you

needed. Now you need to eat enough – but no more.

The reason people put weight back on is that they start eating too much for their needs (often reverting to their old eating habits) and aren't active enough. Pure and simple. So here we look at the practical ways to stop this from happening, and then on pages 178–9 we examine the factors other than true hunger or need that make you eat too much, and show you how to recognise them.

Eat to Suit Your Lifestyle and Yourself

One of the main points of this book – offering several different ways to lose weight – is that I recognise the importance of a plan that you like. Our participants lost weight successfully because their chosen plans fitted in with their lifestyles and their tastes. Neither are the plans too restricted on calories. Both these factors mean that you already have a head start in maintaining your new weight. You don't need to feel that you've 'finished the diet' and now you have to eat differently again. The six plans can each be used as a base on which to build your maintenance diet, which is explained below.

Don't Aim Too Low!

After your six-week programme is up, you have two choices. Either you carry on slimming, or you begin a maintenance programme.

If you are still overweight, you can use the programme for a further few weeks or as long as necessary to get down to a sensible weight for you. However, it is vital to your long-term success in keeping the weight off that you don't aim for too low a weight. Aim too low and you will need to eat too little in order to maintain it – and in any case, too thin has almost as many health risks as too fat. So aim for a reasonable weight. Work out your current Body Mass Index, measure your waist circumference and follow all the other guidelines in Chapters 1 and 2 to decide if your new weight *is* reasonable. If the answer is 'yes', rather than saying, 'Great, the diet's finished, I can eat what I want now', you need to gradually build up your calorie intake to a maintenance level.

Up Your Calorie Intake Gradually

You may remember that I explained how in the first week or two of going on a reduced-calorie diet, you lose several pounds which aren't body fat, but a mix of fluid and glycogen, thus explaining the rapid weight loss that then slows down.

At the end of a period of eating to slim, if you suddenly up your calorie intake you will find that the glycogen/fluid rapidly returns and you will hop on the scales and find that you seem to have put on 3 lb or so overnight. This *isn't* fat, but it is still demoralising. To avoid this happening, it is best to take two or three weeks gradually to increase your calorie intake. The glycogen gain will still happen, slowly, but over those weeks you will still be losing a little body fat which will go some way towards compensating.

Week 1 Pre-maintenance

I suggest that you simply increase your calorie intake by having two extra small snacks a day, adding up to 200 more calories a day. Choose these from the various snack lists within the six slimming plans, or from the charts at the end of this chapter, and try to make them nutritious – bread, nuts, seeds, fruit, etc.

Week 2 Pre-maintenance

I suggest that as well as the extra snacks, you increase portion sizes of the carbohydrate element of your main meals very slightly – an extra couple of spoonfuls of potato or rice, say, with your main meal, plus an extra slice of bread with your breakfast or lunch. This will add about another 200 calories a day, so by the end of Week 2 you will have added 400 calories to your diet. Most of the diets (for women) are based on 1,300 calories a day, so that means your intake will be 1,700 now.

Week 3 Maintenance

From Week 3 onwards, you can follow a long-term maintenance diet, increasing calories again by another 200–300 (depending upon your own metabolic rate and how much exercise you do). This can easily be taken up by increasing the portion size of your main meal slightly – say, a bit more protein such as meat, fish, pulses, and a little more carbohydrate again, plus allowing yourself, say, 100 calories' worth of some kind of food or drink you especially enjoy – a glass of wine or beer, or a piece of chocolate.

So this is how your calorie intake will look now (for women):

Your basic diet – same as six-week plan	1,300 calories
Extra snack foods	200 calories
Larger portion sizes	300–400 calories
Treat	100 calories
Total	1,900–2,000 calories a day

(Men should have larger portions again at each meal, say 3 × 200 calories extra which will bring them to a reasonable daily total for males of 2,500–2,600.)

You will see that in getting your calorie intake back up to a maintenance level, I haven't suggested that you alter your eating patterns from what they were while you were losing weight – we've simply increased calories in a sensible, balanced way.

And that is how you need to eat to maintain your new weight. On a varied and nutritious diet that keeps fat levels reasonable and that will help you to develop a long-term taste for good food, and a long-term habit of keeping the less useful calories down to a minimum. Of course, you can't carry on using any one six-week plan for the rest of your life – this is just an outline of how you could eat. You can use the charts at the end of this chapter to devise your own healthy meals.

Success on snacks

Eating 'little and often' is an excellent principle to follow to help you keep slim. This helps to keep hunger pangs at bay, helps you to avoid bingeing, gives your mouth something to do frequently, and helps your digestive system. But make sure that most of your snacks are healthy ones – mini meals, or things like fresh fruit, dried fruit, seeds, nuts, cereals, bread.

Using the charts

The food charts on pages 182–8 show you the calories and fat in what you are eating. One of the most interesting things that they show is the percentage of fat, carbohydrate and protein in what you eat. An ideal percentage breakdown in the diet for the three major nutrients (and suppliers of calories) is about 30 per cent fat, about 15 per cent protein and about 55 per cent carbohydrate. So if the majority of the foods that you eat contain the fat, protein and carbohydrates in roughly these proportions, you can be sure you are getting a reasonably healthy diet.

These percentage figures won't match what you will find on food labels. That is because when a commercial food label says something like, 'only 5 per cent fat', what it means is fat by weight – i.e. 5g out of every 100g of the product are fat grams. But, because the majority of the weight of food is water – even seemingly solid things like cheese (36 per cent water), or lean meat (74 per cent water) or potatoes (79 per cent water) – which contains no calories or major nutrients, the true percentage of fat as a proportion of the nutrients in the food will be much larger.

To give an example, minced meat may carry a label saying 'extra lean, less than 8 per cent fat' – i.e. no more than 8g of fat per 100g of product. There are 188 calories in 100g of product. Each gram of fat contains 9 calories, therefore there are up to 72 fat calories in 100g of product. This works out at a true figure of 38 per cent fat in the product as a percentage of total nutrients.

If you are watching your fat intake – which, because fat is higher in calories than any other nutrient, is a good idea for long-term weight control – it is this 'real' percentage that you need to know.

Exercise

As we've seen, to maintain your new weight you need to maintain the energy balance. Continuing with a regular exercise programme is probably the single most important thing you can do to help that balance.

You've been burning 250 calories a day 'extra' to help you lose an additional half pound or so a week. As 3,500 calories burnt is equivalent to a pound of body fat burnt when you're slimming, it is also equivalent to a pound of body fat not gained when you're maintaining weight.

If you did your '250' just three times a week, over the course of a year that would represent 39,000 calories or just over 11 lb of fat that you haven't put on. Do it four times a week, that would be 15 lbs' worth of calories that you've burnt. In other words – exercise helps you stay slim, in a big way. Looked at another way, it allows you to eat more than you would be able to if you did no exercise, without putting on weight.

And lastly, if you need more encouragement, look back to pages 164–6 and all the other many benefits of exercise. So please, do keep up with your activity and enjoy it for all the plus points it will bring you.

Food for Thought – Why You Eat What You Eat

What makes you overeat – apart from genuine hunger and need? Most of us, I estimate, eat between a quarter and a half more food and drink than our bodies actually need, for sustenance.

The five main non-hunger reasons to eat are Habit, Food Promotion, Comfort, Boredom and Sociability, and between them I think they have a lot to answer for. They are the real reason most of us put on weight and find it hard to shift; why many of us put back on lost weight; and why keeping a good shape seems like a permanent battle. If we only ate when we felt hungry or needed particular nutrients, there would be no problem.

If you aren't sure you have been wasting calories on the Fickle Five, try my little questionnaire here. Answer the five sets of questions and tick the box every time you answer yes. If you tick more than one or two boxes in any set, then that non-hunger reason to eat does apply to you and you have been wasting calories. Some of you will probably tick all five boxes in all the Fickle Five. The higher your score, the more important it is that you come to terms with these non-hunger reasons to eat. Self-knowledge is one of the greatest weapons you have when it comes to your weight, and my guidelines below will help you to form a strategy that will work for you.

Habit

☐ Do you eat certain things at certain times of day, most days of the week (e.g. biscuits with morning coffee)?

☐ When you do your regular weekly shop for food are you likely to buy the same items every week with little variation?

☐ When you go to a particular place is it linked in your mind with eating, perhaps even a particular food (e.g. on your regular visit to the garden centre, you always have a scone and a cup of cappuccino)?

☐ Are certain people that you know linked with your eating or drinking a particular item (e.g. when your sister comes round to visit you, you always share a pizza and wine)?

☐ When you go out to buy a non-food item, do you usually buy a food item as well (e.g. you buy a newspaper and pick up a bar of chocolate at the same time)?

Food Promotion

☐ When watching TV, If you see adverts for tempting snacks or food, does it make you go and find something to eat for yourself?

- ☐ When in the supermarket, are you likely to be tempted with '25 per cent extra free' offers on food and 'buy one get one free' promotions?
- ☐ When you go shopping for food, do you always buy more items than you intended?
- ☐ Do you often find that the smell or sight of food makes you buy/eat even if you hadn't been thinking about food before?
- ☐ Do you like to try new foods (e.g. a new flavour yogurt or a new type of biscuit) when they come out?

Comfort

- ☐ Do you turn to food when you have had an argument with someone?
- ☐ Do you find yourself eating when someone has let you down and you feel disappointed or miserable?
- ☐ If you receive a letter telling you that you have not got the job you wanted, or failed the exam, will a coffee or tea and some biscuits be the way you are most likely to cheer yourself up?
- ☐ If you are having an evening in instead of going out because a friend has let you down, do you tend to eat more than usual?
- ☐ If you are having a hard time at work do you tend to eat more snacks?

Boredom

- ☐ If you miss your train home, will you buy a chocolate bar or muffin to help while away the time until the next one?
- ☐ Are you in a job that you no longer enjoy and find that you're putting on weight?
- ☐ If you're waiting for a special phone call and the call doesn't come, do you pass the time with a pack of biscuits?
- ☐ If you have to do some tedious writing chore at home in the evening, do you find it less irksome if you have a bag of sweets, or similar, to hand?

- ☐ You're in a deadly marriage, nothing in common with your partner, and would leave but for the kids. Do you think that you've been eating more since your marriage began to lose its charm?

Sociability

- ☐ You've eaten before you go to a party. When you get there you find there is a special buffet laid on. Do you eat it anyway?
- ☐ A friend turns up at your house mid morning and you make her coffee. You offer her cake/biscuits. Even though you're not hungry, will you feel obliged to join her in snacking?
- ☐ Someone at the office has a birthday and a cake is cut. Do you say yes to your piece, even though you've just had lunch?
- ☐ You're invited out to a private dinner. The host is over-generous with portion sizes and courses. Do you eat everything that is on your plate at each course?
- ☐ In a restaurant, do you always eat the bread that's offered, and the free peanuts in your local wine bar?

If you answered 'yes' to lots of these questions, read on for some new ways of looking at your eating life …

Kicking the habit

If you ticked several of the 'habit' questions, you eat more than you need without even thinking about what you're doing. Maybe your life is so busy that you just don't register what or when you eat; or maybe you are insecure and find that particular food habits make you feel better. Perhaps you find food shopping and cooking boring, so you do the same old things in the same old ways because it's quicker.

It's time to look at your habits in detail. The best thing you can do is start a food diary, listing everything you eat and drink for a week, and every time you eat a food or a snack or a meal through habit rather than inputting some new thoughts into the process, make a note next to it. Just making a diary will make you 100 per cent more aware of your 'habit foods'. If these happen to be high-fat, high-sugar, high-calorie foods, consider what you can do either to avoid the 'habit' situations (e.g. instead of going to the garden centre mid-morning, why not go as soon as they open so you won't be tempted?) or keep the situations but invest new habits in them (e.g. have something to eat or drink at the garden centre mid-morning but have it instead of breakfast at home; or instead of having fattening gateau, go for something a bit less calorific).

Don't be a fool for food promotions

It's hard, these days, to escape the attentions of the food promoters – the ad men and the huge food manufacturing companies who want you to eat more of their products because it makes them more money. Every time you eat a chocolate bar or a packet cake, part of what you are paying for is the cost of advertising that product.

If you resent that idea, don't buy it. Every time you watch the TV adverts and find yourself with hunger pangs at the sight of an actor tucking into a new brand of pizza, even though you've only just eaten – realise that the big boys of advertising know exactly what they are doing; they spend a fortune researching what makes you want food.

And in the shops, when you succumb to the double pack of chocolate biscuit bars because the extra only costs 50 per cent more – think again. These biscuits won't last you twice as long as the single pack would have done. Because you've bought double at a cheap price, you'll eat them more quickly.

Be aware of what these professionals are doing to get your tastebuds working. That is your best defence against them. Eat when **YOU** want to eat – not when faceless other people want you to eat. Buy what **YOU** want to buy – not what's on someone else's agenda.

Cold comfort

'Comfort eating' is such a well-known phrase because so many people do it. When you're angry, miserable, depressed, tense – you eat. Often, fatty, sweet things. Or you drink – alcohol, which is almost as fattening as fat.

What should you do instead? Well, long term you need to sort out the reasons why you are feeling negative emotions. If you feel a certain way – say, tense – a lot of the time, there must be a root cause. Find the cause and try to do something about it. Hate your job? Hate your boss? Trying to juggle home/work? Then sit down and sort out ways to make things better. It's not just surplus weight that is at stake here, of course – but your own long-term well-being. It is a rare problem for which there isn't a solution or, at least, a compromise. Could also be that you're angry with yourself – you know you should really leave that dead-end job, or whatever, but you haven't been able to work up the guts to move. Take a chance, and put food back in its proper place.

Short term you need a few foolproof strategies for those moments when your hand reaches, with a life of its own, into the biscuit barrel because it knows you are miserable. The easiest strategy is to make sure that the hand finds the barrel is bare – you didn't buy any biscuits (or whatever your best comforter is). It becomes a conscious thing if you have to go down to the shop to find what your hand wants to grab.

You also need an alternative to cheer you up. When you are feeling strong and up, think of five things you can do instead. Picture yourself in the place where you usually feel miserable – say, home, or the office. What can you do there instead? Phone someone who knows you inside-out for a chat? Get your partner to give you a neck massage? Pick some flowers or rerun a favourite comedy video?

Beating boredom

Boredom is really just empty time to fill and you're not sure how to do it. You know the scene. You're hanging around waiting for someone, or there's some other unavoidable delay. Or you get somewhere early. Perhaps someone cancels at the last minute and after being all keyed up you have a spare few hours. Worst of all – everyone else in the home has gone out somewhere exciting and there you are, with nothing but bad movies on TV.

Whether or not you're hungry, food can seem like the most interesting thing on the horizon.

Strange, isn't it, that when you're really busy with no time for yourself at all, dashing around and doing a hundred tasks at once, and hardly any time even to catch up on sleep, you long for a bit of peace and quiet. Time for yourself. When you get it unexpectedly, you don't know what to do with it.

So every time a thought pops into your head about what you'd love to do if only you had the time, write it down. When the spare hour or so arrives, don't be bored – check out the list. Here are some of mine: looking through old photos (who hasn't got stacks?) and maybe making them into an album; starting on that book I've had since goodness knows when; sorting out my wardrobe once and for all and deciding what it needs to revamp it; writing letters to friends; phoning friends; taking cuttings from my houseplants.

Obviously you can't do most of those waiting for a train or sitting on a bus – but you could always make sure you carry something with you to read. A book is, really, all you ever need to beat boredom. If you choose well it's better than TV. So plan ahead and if you can't afford to buy, join the library.

Sociable sense

It is, let's face it, terribly, terribly easy to overeat and drink excessively if you lead a busy social life.

Surprisingly, it is also quite easy **NOT** to.

However, you do need to be very aware of the potential for dietary disaster every time you are out and about, entertaining, or with friends. If this is your major problem out of the 'Fickle Five', you have probably followed the Business Plan, within which there were plenty of tips on reducing your calorie intake while eating out or entertaining. Here are a few more thoughts you may like to digest (calorie-free).

I think that avoiding social calories, over and above what you need for true sustenance, comes down to one decision. Do you want to be slim? Or do you want to eat and drink whatever you want whenever you want and be overweight? Which is most important to you?

If you choose the former, then you simply learn to spot the traps and say no when one comes along. Again, planning ahead is an excellent strategy. If you know you are going out to the pub with friends tonight, eat something sensible before you go and practise saying 'no' to snacks. Decide how many drinks you are going to have and it'll be easier to stick to.

Everywhere you go, if food or drink is offered, ask yourself, Do I really need this? If I say no, will I truly offend anyone? Usually the answer is no, you won't. If you need an alibi, make sure people know beforehand that you are on a special no-alcohol/no added fat/no sugar/no salt (or whatever) diet because of a suspect allergy/digestive problem (or whatever), and let that be your reason to say no to alcohol, cake, crisps or whatever you are being offered.

It's so easy to force hundreds of unwanted calories on your body in minutes. It takes a lot of work to get them off afterwards. Learn to say no to food you don't want. Keep thinking of all the motivators for staying slim. All the reasons you don't want to be fat. If you're going to stay slim for life, you need to want it more than the food. You do, don't you?

Food Charts

For more information on reading these charts see page 177.

* = foods high in sugar, to be limited
    to 10 per cent of total diet.
† = alcohol, similar to carbohydrate
    and contains 7 calories per g.
tr = trace

Food	% Fat	% Carbohydrate	% Protein	Cals/portion	Grams fat/portion	Vitamins	Minerals
Biscuits and bars (all per biscuit or bar)							
Digestive, one large	40	52*	8	75	3.3	...	...
Digestive, choc, small	44	50.5*	5.5	85	4.1	...	...
Gingernut	30	65*	5	45	1.5	...	...
Rich Tea	38.5	56*	5.5	35	1.5	...	...
Shortcake (oblong)	46.5	48.5*	5	75	3.8	...	...
Breads and Crispbreads (all per 25g/1 oz unless otherwise stated)							
Brown	9	75	16	56	0.55	B	...
Cream cracker, one	33	58	9	40	1.5	...	...
French, white	1.2	83.3	15.5	62.5	tr	D	calcium
Meat loaf	12	74.5	13.5	62	0.82	...	iron
Oatcake, one	37	53.5	9.5	45	1.8	...	...
Pitta, white, one	4	82.5	13.5	175	0.8	...	calcium
Pitta, brown, one	7	72	21	160	1.2	...	...
Rice cake, one	7	85.5	7.5	24	0.2	...	...
Ryvita, one	11.5	77.5	11	25	0.2	..	...
Wheatgerm (e.g. Hovis)	8.5	74.5	17	57	0.55	B-group, E	iron
White	6.5	80	13.5	58	0.5	...	calcium, iron
Wholemeal	11	73	16	54	0.67	B-group	iron
Wholemeal bap, one	11	73	16	120	1.5	B-group	iron
Breakfast cereals (all per 25g /1 oz unless otherwise stated)							
All-Bran Plus	18.5	59	22.5	68	1.5	Mos\t	calcium, iron
Branflakes	5.5	76	12.5	80	0.5	C, D, B-group	iron
Cornflakes	4	86.5	9.5	92	0.4	B-group, D	iron
Fruit'n Fibre	12	78	10	90	1.25	B-group, D	iron
Muesli (no added sugar)	19	71	10	82	1.7	E, B3	calcium, iron
Porridge oats, raw	22	63.5	14.5	94	2.25	...	iron
Porridge made up with water, per 100ml	18	70	12	44	0.9	...	iron
Puffed Wheat	3.5	79	17.5	81	0.3	...	...
Shredded Wheat, one	8.5	78.5	13	80	0.75	...	...
Special K	6	75.5	18.5	97	0.6	B-group, D	iron
Weetabix, one	9	77.5	13.5	65	0.65	B3	iron
Cakes and Bakery items (all per item or slice)							
Chocolate, rich, small slice (50g /2 oz)	53	42*	5	230	13.6	...	...
Croissant, one (65g)	54	38.5	7.5	280	16.5	...	...
Crumpet, one	3.5	83	13.5	100	0.5	...	calcium, iron
Doughnut, jam, one	41	52.5	6.5	260	12	...	...
Eclair, chocolate, one	57.5	38*	4.5	190	12	...	...
Rich fruit cake, small slice (50g /2 oz)	30	66*	4	165	5.5	A	iron
Scone, plain, one	35.5	56.5*	8	200	8	...	...
Victoria sponge, one slice (50g /2 oz)	51.5	43*	5.5	230	13.25	...	...
Cheese (all per 25g /1 oz unless otherwise stated)							
Brie or Camembert	69.5	tr	30.5	75	5.8	A, B-group, D	calcium
Cheddar	74.5	tr	25.5	101	8.3	A, B-group, D	calcium
Cheddar-style, half fat	50.5	tr	49.5	62	3.5	A, B-group, D	calcium
Cheese spread	73	1	26	71	5.7	A, B-group, D	calcium

Food	% Fat	% Carbohydrate	% Protein	Cals/portion	Grams fat/portion	Vitamins	Minerals
Cottage cheese, diet	18	tr	82	20	0.4	B₂	calcium
Cottage cheese, standard	37.5	5.5	57	24	1.0	B₂	calcium
Cream cheese, full fat	97	tr	3	110	12	A	...
Danish Blue	74	tr	26	89	7.3	A, B-group, D	calcium
Edam	68	tr	32	76	5.7	A, B-group, D	calcium
Mozzarella, Italian	68	3	29	62	4.75	...	calcium
Soft cheese, low-fat	57	7.5	35.5	33	2.1	...	calcium
Stilton	78	tr	22	115	10	A, B-group, D	calcium

Dressings, Sauces and Pickles (all per tbsp)

	% Fat	% Carbohydrate	% Protein	Cals/portion	Grams fat/portion	Vitamins	Minerals
Brown sauce	tr	95.5*	4.5	20	tr	...	...
Burger relish	tr	98	2	21	tr	...	...
French dressing	100	tr	tr	130	14.5	...	...
Mayonnaise	99	tr	1	143	15.75	...	...
Salad cream	79	18*	3	62	5.5	...	...
Soy sauce	6	71	23	11	tr	...	...
Sweet pickle	2	96*	2	26	tr	...	...
Tomato ketchup	1	91*	8	20	tr	...	...

Drinks

Alcoholic drinks

	% Fat	% Carbohydrate	% Protein	Cals/portion	Grams fat/portion	Vitamins	Minerals
Beer, (275ml/½ pint)	tr	96.5†	3.5	90	tr	...	...
Lager, (275ml/½ pint)	tr	97.5†	2.5	90	tr	...	...
Port, (25ml/1 fl oz)	...	100†	tr	40	tr	...	...
Sherry, (25ml/1 fl oz)	...	100†	tr	30	...	...	...
Spirits, all, 1 measure	...	100†	...	50	...	...	...
Stout, (275ml/½ pint)	tr	100†	tr	90	tr	...	...
Wine, red, (140ml/5 fl oz)	...	99†	1	100	...	...	...
Wine, white, medium, (140ml/5 fl oz)	...	100†	...	100	...	...	...
Wine, white dry, (140ml/5 fl oz)	...	100†	...	90	...	...	...
Wine, white, sweet, (140ml/5 fl oz)	...	99†	1	140	...	...	...

Beverages

	% Fat	% Carbohydrate	% Protein	Cals/portion	Grams fat/portion	Vitamins	Minerals
Tea	...	tr	tr	tr	...	...	...
Coffee, one tspn	...	41	59	2.5	...	...	...
Hot chocolate, per 200ml/7 fl oz	19	69*	12	112	2.4	B₃	calcium
Low-calorie instant hot chocolate, per sachet	24	56*	20	40	1	...	...

Soft drinks

	% Fat	% Carbohydrate	% Protein	Cals/portion	Grams fat/portion	Vitamins	Minerals
Cola, 1 × 330ml/12 fl oz can	...	100*	...	135	...	...	...
Lemonade, one 200ml/7 fl oz glass	...	100*	...	50	...	...	...
Orange squash, one 200ml/7 fl oz glass	...	100*	...	60	...	...	...

Fruit juices (all per average 125ml/4½ fl oz glass)

	% Fat	% Carbohydrate	% Protein	Cals/portion	Grams fat/portion	Vitamins	Minerals
Apple	...	97	3	50	...	...	...
Grape	...	97	3	75	...	...	...
Grapefruit	...	96	4	50	...	C	...
Mixed citrus	...	96	4	50	...	C	...
Mixed vegetable	...	85	15	25	...	C	...
Orange	...	95	5	50	...	C	...
Pineapple	...	97	3	55	...	C	...
Tomato	...	83	17	25	...	C	...

Eggs

	% Fat	% Carbohydrate	% Protein	Cals/portion	Grams fat/portion	Vitamins	Minerals
Size 2 (large), one egg	67	tr	33	90	6.8	A, B-group, D, E	calcium, iron
Size 3 (medium), one egg	67	tr	33	80	6	A, B-group, D, E	calcium, iron
Size 4 (small), one egg	67	tr	33	75	5.5	A, B-group, D, E	calcium, iron
Size 3 (medium), fried, drained	78	tr	22	120	10.5	A, B-group, D, E	calcium, iron
Size 3 (medium), scrambled with 7g/¼ oz low-fat spread and 25ml/1 fl oz skimmed milk)	64	4	32	115	9	A, B-group, D, E	calcium, iron

Food	% Fat	% Carbohydrate	% Protein	Cals/portion	Grams fat/portion	Vitamins	Minerals
Fats and Oils (all per 25g (1 oz))							
Butter	100	tr	tr	185	20.5	A, D	...
Low-fat spread	100	...	...	91	10	A, D	...
Margarine, all types, including sunflower	100	tr	tr	182	20.3	A, D	...
Oils, all kinds	100	...	tr	225	25	...	...
Very low-fat spread	100	...	...	57	6.3	A, D	...
Fish and Seafood (all per 100g/3$\frac{1}{2}$ oz unless otherwise stated)							
Cod, coley, haddock or monkfish fillet	8	...	92	76	0.7	B$_3$	calcium
Deep-fried fish in batter	47	14	39	200	10.3	...	...
Fish finger, grilled, one	38	34	28	50	2	...	...
Fish, frozen, in light batter, baked or grilled, one portion (100g/3$\frac{1}{2}$ oz)	51.5	28.5	20	203	11.6	...	...
Haddock, smoked fillet	8	...	92	100	0.9	B-group	calcium
Herring, fillet	71	...	29	234	18.5	B-group, D	calcium, iron
Kipper, grilled fillet	50	...	50	205	11.4	A, B-group, D	calcium, iron
Pilchards in tomato sauce	38.5	2	59.5	126	5.4	B-group, D, E	calcium
Plaice, fillet	18	...	82	93	1.9	B-group	calcium
Salmon, fresh fillet	59	...	41	197	13	A, B-group, D	...
Salmon, pink, canned	47.5	...	52.5	155	8.2	A, B-group, D, E	calcium, iron
Salmon, smoked	28.5	...	71.5	142	4.5	A, B-group, D	...
Scampi, deep-fried	50	34	16	316	17.6	...	calcium, iron
Trout, one average (225g/8 oz)	30	...	70	200	6.75	B$_3$	iron
Tuna in brine, drained	3	...	97	114	0.35	B-group	iron
Tuna in oil, drained	47	...	53	210	11	B-group, E	iron
Whitebait, deep-fried	81	4	15	525	47.5	...	calcium, iron
Seafood							
Crabmeat	37	...	63	127	5.2	B-group	calcium
Crabmeat, canned	10	...	90	81	0.9	...	calcium, iron
Mussels, shelled	20.5	tr	79.5	87	2	...	calcium, iron
Prawns, shelled	15	...	85	107	1.8	B-group	calcium
Scallops, shelled	12	tr	88	105	1.4	...	calcium, iron
Squid	15	tr	85	82	1.4	A, B$_3$	calcium, iron
Fruit (all per item, unless otherwise stated)							
Apple, dessert	tr	97	3	45	tr	...	...
Apple, cooking, per 25g/1 oz	tr	97	3	40	tr	...	...
Apricot, fresh	tr	93	7	10	tr	A	...
Apricots, dried, per 25g/1 oz	tr	89.5	10.5	45	tr	A	...
Banana, medium	3.5	91	5.5	80	0.3	A, C, E	...
Blackberries, 25g/1 oz	tr	83	17	7	tr	C	calcium, iron
Blackcurrants, 25g/1 oz	tr	88	12	7	tr	C	calcium, iron
Currants, dried 25g/1 oz	tr	97	3	60	tr	...	...
Cherries, 25g/1 oz	tr	95	5	10	tr	...	...
Damsons, 25g/1 oz	tr	95	5	8	tr	...	...
Dates, each, fresh or dry	tr	96.5	3.5	15	tr	...	iron
Dates, stoned, 25g/1 oz	tr	96.5	3.5	62	tr	...	iron
Fig, dry	tr	93	7	53	tr	...	iron
Fig, fresh	tr	87	13	10	tr	...	iron
Gooseberries, cooking, per 25g/1 oz	tr	93	7	9	tr	C, E	...
Gooseberries, dessert, per 25g/1 oz	tr	75	25	4	tr	C, E	...
Grapefruit, half	tr	90	10	20	tr	C	...
Kiwi fruit	6	86	8	25	tr	C	...
Lemon	tr	80	20	15	tr	C	...
Lime	tr	80	20	10	tr	C	...
Mango	tr	97	3	100	tr	C, A	iron
Melon, 200g/7 oz slice	tr	90	10	25	tr	A, C	...
Nectarine	tr	93	7	50	tr	A, B$_3$	...
Orange	tr	92	8	50	tr	C	calcium

Food	% Fat	% Carbohydrate	% Protein	Cals/portion	Grams fat/portion	Vitamins	Minerals
Peach	tr	92	8	50	tr	A	...
Pear, medium	tr	98	2	50	tr	...	...
Pineapple, one ring	tr	95	5	25	tr	C	...
Plum, one dessert	tr	94	6	20	tr	...	...
Prunes, each	tr	94	6	10	tr	A	iron
Prunes, stoned per 25g/1 oz	tr	94	6	40	tr	A	iron
Raisin, 25g/1 oz	tr	98	2	61	tr	...	...
Raspberries, 25g/1 oz	tr	84	16	6	tr	C	iron
Rhubarb, one large stick, 100g/3½ oz	tr	62.5	37.5	6	tr	C	calcium
Satsuma or tangerine	tr	91	9	20	tr	C	...
Strawberries, 25g/1 oz	tr	90	10	6	tr	C	iron
Sultanas, 25g/1 oz	tr	97	3	62	tr	...	iron

Grains (all per 25g/1 oz unless otherwise stated)

Food	% Fat	% Carbohydrate	% Protein	Cals/portion	Grams fat/portion	Vitamins	Minerals
Flour, white	3	86	11	87	0.3	...	calcium, iron
Flour, wholemeal	6	77.5	16.5	80	0.5	B₃	iron
Pasta, brown (boiled weight)	8.5	72.5	18	32	0.3	...	iron
Pasta, brown, all shapes (dry weight)	7	78	15	85	0.6	...	iron
Pasta, white (boiled weight)	3	83	14	29	tr	...	iron
Pasta, white, all shapes (dry weight)	3	83	14	95	0.25	...	iron
Pearl barley (dry weight)	4	87	9	90	0.4	...	...
Rice, brown (boiled weight)	7	86	7	30	0.45	B-group, E	iron
Rice, brown (dry weight)	7	85	6	90	0.7	B-group, E	iron
Rice, white (boiled weight)	2	90	8	30	tr	...	iron
Rice, white (dry weight)	2.5	90	7.5	90	0.25	...	iron
Rice salad (ready-made)	13	75	12	35	0.5	...	...
Spaghetti in tomato sauce, 213g/7½ oz can	10.5	77.5	12	127	1.5	...	iron

Meat and Poultry (all per 25g/1 oz unless otherwise stated)

Food	% Fat	% Carbohydrate	% Protein	Cals/portion	Grams fat/portion	Vitamins	Minerals
Bacon, back, trimmed, grilled	58	...	42	73	4.7	B₃	...
Bacon, streaky, grilled	77	...	23	105	9	B₃	...
Beef, minced	60	...	40	57	3.8	B-group	iron
Beef, minced, extra-lean	35	...	65	47	1.8	B-group	iron
Beef, roast, lean only	25	...	75	40	1.1	B-group	iron
Beef steak, lean only, grilled	32	...	68	42	1.5	B-group	iron
Beefburger, one 50g/2 oz frozen burger, grilled	64	5	31	120	8.5	B-group	iron
Chicken, average breast with skin, 200g/7 oz grilled	60	...	40	225	15	B-group	iron
Chicken, average breast without skin, 200g/7 oz grilled	42	...	58	150	7	B-group	iron
Chicken fillet, no skin, raw	30	...	70	30	1	B-group	iron
Chicken, roast, meat only	33	...	67	37	1.3	B-group	iron
Corned beef	50	...	50	54	3	B-group, E	iron
Duck, breast fillet	46	...	54	47	2.4	B₃	iron
Duck, roast, meat and skin	77	...	23	85	7.2	B₃	iron
Gammon steak, grilled, lean only	27	...	73	43	1.3	B₁, B₃	iron
Ham, extra lean	37.5	...	62.5	30	1.25	B₃	...
Kidneys, lamb's	27	...	73	22	0.67	A, B-group, E	iron
Lamb, one average trimmed chop	50	...	50	120	6.8	B₃	iron
Lamb, leg, roast, lean only	38	...	62	48	2	B₃	iron
Lamb, shoulder, roast	75	...	25	80	6.5	B₃	iron
Liver, lamb's	52	3	45	45	2.5	A, B-group, E	iron
Liver sausage	78	5.5	16.5	77	6.7	B-group	iron
Luncheon meat, canned pork	77.5	6.5	16	78	6.7	...	...
Pork, fillet, raw	43	...	57	37	1.75	B₃	iron
Pork, roast, lean only	34	...	66	46	1.7	B₃	iron
Rabbit (excl. bone)	29	...	71	31	1	B₃, B₁₂	iron
Salami	83	1	16	122	11.3	B₃	...
Sausages, beef, grilled, per chipolata	59	21.5	19.5	70	4.5	B₃, E	iron
Sausages, low-fat grilled, per chipolata	43	23	34	50	2.4	B₃, E	iron
Sausages, pork, grilled, per chipolata	70	13.5	16.5	75	5.8	B₃, E	iron

Food	% Fat	% Carbohydrate	% Protein	Cals/portion	Grams fat/portion	Vitamins	Minerals
Turkey, dark meat (no skin)	28	...	72	28	0.9	B-group	iron
Turkey, light meat (no skin)	9.5	...	90.5	26	0.3	B-group	iron
Tongue	70	...	30	53	4	B-group	iron
Veal, fillet, raw	22	...	78	27	0.6	B-group	iron
Venison, fillet	29	...	71	49	1.6	B$_3$	iron

Milk and Cream (all per 25g/1 fl oz unless otherwise stated)

Food	% Fat	% Carbohydrate	% Protein	Cals/portion	Grams fat/portion	Vitamins	Minerals
Instant, low-fat milk, dry, per tbsp	3	56	41	18	tr	D	calcium
Milk, whole	52.5	27	20.5	16	1	A, B-group	calcium
Milk, semi-skimmed	31.5	39	29.5	11.5	0.4	B-group	calcium
Milk, skimmed	2	57	41	8	tr	B-group	calcium
Soya milk	53.5	10	36.5	8	0.5	D	calcium
Aerosol cream	87	10	3	16	1.5	...	calcium
Double cream	97	1.5	1.5	112	12	D	calcium
Single cream	90	5.5	4.5	53	5.3	D	calcium
Sour cream	88	7	5	51	5	D	calcium

Nuts and Crisps (all per 25g/1 oz shelled weight)

Food	% Fat	% Carbohydrate	% Protein	Cals/portion	Grams fat/portion	Vitamins	Minerals
Almonds	85	3	12	141	13.3	E	calcium
Brazils	89.5	2.5	8	155	15.3	E	calcium
Chestnuts	14	81	5	42	0.67	...	...
Hazelnuts	85	7	8	95	9	E	...
Peanuts, fresh or dry-roasted	77.5	5.5	17	142	12.2	E, B$_3$	...
Walnuts	89	3	8	131	9	...	...
Crisps, standard	60.5	34.5	5	133	9	...	...
Lower-fat crisps	56	36.5	7.5	105	6.5	...	...

Pastry and Pizza

Food	% Fat	% Carbohydrate	% Protein	Cals/portion	Grams fat/portion	Vitamins	Minerals
Cornish pasty, one small (130g/4½ oz)	55.5	35	9.5	430	26.5	...	...
Filo, (25g/1 oz)	9.5	78	12.5	67	0.7	...	...
Flaky, (25g/1 oz)	64.5	31.5	4	106	7.6	...	...
Jam tart, one	35	61	4	150	5.8	...	...
Mince pie, one	43	53	4	200	9.5	...	...
Pork pie, one individual, (140g/5 oz)	64.5	25	10.5	530	37.8	B$_3$	iron
Quiche, one slice, (100g/3½ oz)	65	20	15	390	28	A	calcium, iron
Sausage roll, 1 large	68	26	6	270	20.5	...	...
Shortcrust, (25g/1 oz)	55	40	5	113	7	...	...
Steak and kidney, one individual (130g/4½ oz)	59	30	11	480	31.5	A, B$_{12}$	iron

Puddings and Desserts

Food	% Fat	% Carbohydrate	% Protein	Cals/portion	Grams fat/portion	Vitamins	Minerals
Black Forest gateau (per 100g/3½ oz)	53	42*	5	310	18.2	...	...
Cheesecake (per 50g/2 oz portion)	75	21*	4	210	17.5	A	calcium
Custard, ready-made (100ml/3½ oz)	34	53*	13	120	4.5	...	calcium
Fruit pie (per 100g/3½ oz portion)	38	57.5*	4.5	180	7.6	...	...
Ice cream, vanilla (per 50g/2 oz portion)	35.5	55.5*	9	83	3.3	...	calcium
Trifle (per 100g/3½ oz portion)	34	57*	9	160	6.1	A	calcium

Pulses, Beans, Peas and Lentils (all per 25g/1 oz)

Food	% Fat	% Carbohydrate	% Protein	Cals/portion	Grams fat/portion	Vitamins	Minerals
Baked beans in tomato sauce	6	61	33	16	0.1	E	calcium, iron
Butter beans, canned or boiled	2.5	67.5	30	23	tr	E	iron
Chickpeas, canned or boiled	18	60	22	40	0.8	E	iron
Haricot beans, canned or boiled	5	67	28	23	0.1	E	iron
Kidney beans, canned or boiled	4.5	59.5	36	25	0.1	...	iron
Lentils, dry weight	3	65.5	31.5	76	0.25	...	iron
Lentils, boiled	4.5	64.5	31	25	0.1	...	iron
Split peas, boiled	2.5	69.5	28	30	tr	...	iron

Food	% Fat	% Carbohydrate	% Protein	Cals/portion	Grams fat/portion	Vitamins	Minerals
Soups (all per 300g/11 oz serving)							
Cream of chicken	59	29	12	175	11.5	...	...
Cream of tomato	45	46	9	173	8.7	...	...
Lentil	2.5	72.5	25	115	0.3	...	iron
Minestrone	29.5	55	15.5	90	2.9	...	...
Vegetable	14.5	72.5	13	110	1.8	...	...
Spreads (all per 25g/1 oz unless otherwise stated)							
Jam	...	99*	1	65	...	...	...
Liver pâté	67.5	1.5	31	80	6	A, B₁₂	iron
Marmalade	...	100*	tr	65	...	...	...
Marmite, per tsp	3.5	4	92.5	9	tr	B-group	...
Peanut butter	77.5	8	14.5	156	13.4	E, B₃	...
Taramasalata	94	3.5	2.5	110	11.5	...	...
Sugars and Confectionery (all per 25g/1 oz unless otherwise stated)							
Chocolate, milk or plain	51.5	42*	6.5	132	7.5	...	...
Honey	...	99.5*	0.5	72	...	...	...
Sugar	...	100*	...	98	...	...	...
Sugar, per tsp	...	100*	...	20	...	...	...
Sweets, boiled	...	100*	...	82	...	...	...
Syrup	...	100*	...	75	...	...	...
Toffee	36	62*	2	107	4.3	...	...
Vegetables (all per 25g/1 oz unless otherwise stated)							
Artichoke, globe, one whole (edible parts)	1	70	29	15	tr	...	...
Artichoke, Jerusalem	tr	64.5	35.5	4.5	tr	...	...
Asparagus, one spear (50g/2 oz)	tr	24	75.5	4.5	tr	E, C	iron
Aubergine	tr	80	20	3.5	tr	...	...
Avocado, half medium (65g/2½ oz)	89	3	8	145	14.4	E, C	iron
Beans, broad	10.5	55.5	34	12	0.1	A, C, B₃	iron
Beans, French	tr	59	41	10	tr	A	...
Beans, runner	7	53	40	5	tr	A	...
Beansprouts	tr	29	71	7	tr	...	...
Beetroot	tr	84	16	11	tr	...	...
Broccoli	tr	31	69	4.5	tr	A, C, E	calcium, iron
Brussels sprouts	tr	36	62	4.5	tr	A, C, E	...
Cabbage, dark	tr	50	50	6	tr	A, C, E	iron
Cabbage, red	tr	66	34	5	tr	C	calcium
Cabbage, white	tr	65	35	5	tr	C	...
Carrots	tr	88	12	6	tr	A, E	calcium
Cauliflower	tr	42	58	2	tr	C	...
Celery	tr	61	39	2	tr	...	...
Chicory	tr	62	38	2	tr	...	...
Chinese leaves	tr	50	50	3	tr	C, A	iron
Corn on the cob, one	17	70	13	80	1.5	A	...
Courgettes	3.5	67.5	29	5	0.1	A, C	iron
Cucumber	9	67	24	2	tr	...	...
Leek	tr	72	28	8	tr	C, E	calcium, iron
Lettuce	30	37.5	32.5	3	0.1	...	...
Marrow	tr	87	13	4	tr	...	...
Mushrooms	41.5	...	55	3	0.1	...	...
Mustard and cress, whole box	tr	34	64	5	tr	A	...
Onion	tr	85	15	6	tr	C	...
Onion, spring, one	tr	91	9	3	tr	...	...
Parsnip	tr	86.5	13.5	12	tr	E	...
Peas, shelled, fresh or frozen	7	55	38	13	0.1	C	iron
Pepper, green	22.5	53.5	24	4	0.1	A, C, E	...
Pepper, other colours	11	77	12	8	0.1	A, C, E	iron
Potatoes							

Food	% Fat	% Carbohydrate	% Protein	Cals/portion	Grams fat/portion	Vitamins	Minerals
Baked, average (225g/8 oz)	1	89.5	9.5	190	0.2	C	iron
Boiled	1	92	7	20	tr	C	...
Chips, average cut (25g/1 oz)	41.5	55	3.5	65	3	...	...
Chips, oven	32	62.5	5.5	49	1.75	...	...
Instant mash, made up	9.5	79	11.5	16	0.2	C	...
Mashed	38	57	5	30	1.25	C	...
Roast, one chunk (50g/2 oz)	27.5	65	7.5	80	2.4	C	iron
Radish	tr	70	30	4	tr	C	iron
Spinach	14.5	17.5	68	7	0.1	A, C, E	calcium, iron
Swede	tr	77	13	5	tr	C	...
Sweet potato	6.5	88.5	5	21	0.15	A, C, E	...
Sweetcorn kernels	15	69.5	15.5	30	0.5	A	...
Tomato, one average (50g/2 oz)	tr	75	25	7	tr	A, C, E	...
Tomatoes, canned	1	62.5	36.5	3	tr	A, C, E	iron
Turnip	22	62	16	4	0.1	C	calcium, iron
Watercress	tr	17	83	3	tr	A, C	calcium, iron

Vegetarian Products

Food	% Fat	% Carbohydrate	% Protein	Cals/portion	Grams fat/portion	Vitamins	Minerals
Nut loaf (100g/3½ oz)	41	41	18	210	9.5	...	...
Quorn (25g/1 oz)	34	8	58	21	0.8	n/k	n/k
Sosmix, made up (100g/3½ oz)	59	24	17	170	11.2	...	calcium, iron
Tofu, (25g/1 oz)	53	3	44	17	1	...	calcium, iron
TVP mince, reconstituted weight (25g/1 oz)	2.5	39	58.5	17	tr	...	calcium, iron
Vegeburger (50g/2 oz)	45	22.5	32.5	81	4	...	calcium, iron

Yogurt and Fromage Frais (all per 25g/1 oz unless otherwise stated)

Food	% Fat	% Carbohydrate	% Protein	Cals/portion	Grams fat/portion	Vitamins	Minerals
Fromage frais, diet fruit (100g/3½ oz)	2	39.5	58.5	43	0.1	...	calcium
Fromage frais, fruit	27	48*	25	28	0.85	...	calcium
Fromage frais natural (8% fat)	64	9	27	28	2	...	calcium
Fromage frais, natural, very low-fat	4	22	74	12	tr	...	calcium
Yogurt, diet fruit, (125g/4½ oz)	2	54	44	51	0.1	...	calcium
Yogurt, fruit	9.5	70.5*	20	1024	0.25	...	calcium
Yogurt, natural, low-fat	13.5	48	38.5	13	0.25	...	calcium
Yogurt, natural, whole-milk	52	25	23	17	1	...	calcium
Yogurt, strained, Greek	61	n'k	n/k	33	2.25	...	calcium

N/k Not known.

Index

The HEADLINE money-back guarantee for
6 Ways to Lose a Stone in 6 Weeks

Headline is offering a guarantee of weight loss or your money back.

If you fail to lose weight having followed one of the six plans over an entire six-week period and wish to claim your money back, then the following terms and conditions apply:

Terms and conditions:

1. Your copy of *6 Ways to Lose a Stone in 6 Weeks* must be returned to the publisher within 7 weeks of purchase.
2. The till receipt for the book must be sent at time of return along with a short letter stating which plan you tried and why you were dissatisfied.
3. Offer valid until 31 July 1999, i.e. refund requests must arrive with the publishers by this date.
5. Your book, letter and till receipt should be sent to:

Headline Book Publishing
6 Ways Guarantee
338 Euston Road
London
NW1 3BH

6. Refunds will be repaid by cheque within 28 days of receipt.